Life at Full Throttle

Attention Deficit/Hyperactivity Disorder in Adults

Catherine Avery, Ph.D.

iUniverse, Inc.
New York   Bloomington

The information, ideas, and suggestions in this book are not intended as a substitute for professional medical advice. Before following any suggestions contained in this book, you should consult your personal physician. Neither the author nor the publisher shall be liable or responsible for any loss or damage allegedly arising as a consequence of your use or application of any information or suggestions in this book.

iUniverse books may be ordered through booksellers or by contacting:

iUniverse
1663 Liberty Drive
Bloomington, IN 47403
www.iuniverse.com
1-800-Authors (1-800-288-4677)

Because of the dynamic nature of the Internet, any Web addresses or links contained in this book may have changed since publication and may no longer be valid. The views expressed in this work are solely those of the author and do not necessarily reflect the views of the publisher, and the publisher hereby disclaims any responsibility for them.

ISBN: 978-1-4401-9463-4 (sc)
ISBN: 978-1-4401-9461-0 (dj)
ISBN: 978-1-4401-9462-7 (ebook)

Library of Congress Control Number: 2009912442

Printed in the United States of America

iUniverse rev. date: 12/28/09

To my parents, with deepest love and appreciation

Contents

Preface

As an AD/HD adult, I typically skip over the preface section in books. I'm impatient to get to the "real stuff." So in an attempt to remain consistent—a goal that has eluded me for most of my adult life—I think I'll skip this preface as well.

Chapter 1

How I Forgot Santa in the Bathroom

Every AD/HD adult has his or her own story to tell: some parts are painful; some elicit deep regret or unresolved shame. But there are also "AD/HD moments" that are so common to adults with Attention Deficit/Hyperactivity Disorder that, when viewed with the correct mixture of irreverence and humor, provoke gales of laughter, as well as a sense that those of us with AD/HD may actually have a little more fun in this adventure called life—that is, if we allow ourselves to. I have always told my children that when I am old and senile—rocking back and forth on the porch with a toothless grin—I will be in the process of reliving some of the funnier moments of my life. And believe me, I've amassed enough to humor me for years of senility.

In this book I will talk about the AD/HD experience from a unique set of perspectives: as a clinical psychologist who has evaluated more than two thousand AD/HD children and adults over the past fifteen years; as a mother who has parented two children with attentional deficits; and as a woman who has lived with the symptoms of this disorder for as long as she can remember. I have no intention of making excuses for adults with AD/HD, and I believe that identifying and taking ownership of problem behaviors is critical to success. However, I will also not condemn those of us who, despite these efforts, repeatedly fall short of our plans and expectations. There is a middle ground that is composed of compassion, experience, education, and humor that I encourage clients with AD/HD to find, and I hope to maintain this perspective throughout this book.

Because humor is so important in the life of an AD/HD adult, I will start with my finest "AD/HD moment": when I forgot Santa in the bathroom. If the particularly observant reader notices that my AD/

1

HD moment extended for well over a month, let me just say that time is relative in the AD/HD world.

The following story is the truth, the whole truth, and nothing but the truth—at least I think it is. The AD/HD imagination is so fertile and the tendency for AD/HDers to create stimulation is so second nature that it is possible that I've added a bit here and there as I've told this story over the years. Dr. Edward Hallowell, speaking at the first national AD/HD conference for adults,[1] noted that people with AD/HD tend to exaggerate when telling a story and asserted that they shouldn't feel guilty for their penchant to embellish for the sake of entertainment (or stimulation). I have taken this gem of wisdom as blanket permission to let go of years of guilt over the fact that I exaggerate from time to time—particularly if I'm restless … or in a good mood … or in a bad mood … or if I have a particularly engaged audience … or if I'm trying to engage an audience … Hmmm, let's just get back to Santa, okay?

It was November, the beginning of a crazily busy season for those of us who do not plan well, and as PTA president of a local elementary school, I was in charge of organizing a Christmas party to be held immediately following an all-school Christmas concert. Now, there are some people who excel at planning large events like this—first organizing a committee, identifying tasks, and delegating responsibility, and then following through to make certain that the various tasks have been completed. These people that I am describing do not have AD/HD. Most people with AD/HD are wonderful at the initial planning stages where imagination and creativity are a plus. But translating ideas into action requires ongoing coordination with others who seem to function best between the hours of 8:00 am and 8:00 pm. Midnight powwows have not yet caught on in PTA circles, although that's when many people with AD/HD do their best work.

Large projects also typically involve meetings, a concept that sends shivers up the spines of my more hyperactive brethren. In the AD/HD world, the word *meeting* is translated as follows: "An indefinite period of forced captivity, during which time one must try to remain focused while simultaneously stifling the overwhelming desire to interrupt, doodle, or pass humorous notes." The mere prospect of group meetings is often enough to convince AD/HDers that it would be less painful to tackle an entire project by themselves. Initially the idea of "going solo" is met with great enthusiasm and splendid imagery of ultimate success, and memories of disastrous past projects are overshadowed by the excitement of a new venture. So, in true AD/HD form, I decided that there was clearly enough time to plan and execute the party by myself.

To my credit, I had the entire party planned a month ahead of time—in my mind. I would solicit donations from local businesses and make up darling little Christmas goodie bags, one for each elementary school student. The bags would be decorated during art class. The art teacher, of course, would be smitten with this idea, and the final products would be filled with the donated holiday treats and set out on a large table by the entrance to the cafeteria. I had run over this scenario countless times in my mind, imagining little children pulling their parents by the arm, saying, "Come on, Mommy and Daddy! You have to see the bag that I decorated all by myself!" We would have a group of parents bring in homemade desserts, and to top it all off, Santa would arrive in full costume, with a burlap bag filled with candy canes.

The next thing I knew, the concert was a week away, and the series of events that transpired will be only too familiar to those readers with organizational deficiencies. At the risk of precipitating a post-traumatic stress response in my AD/HD comrades, let me share with you the following sequence of events, which began with a great plan and ended with an abandoned Santa Claus. As my husband would say, "What were you thinking?" Do you really want to know? Welcome to the AD/HD world …

How did three weeks slip by? Jeez! There's no way I can ask the art teacher to take on the bags as a Christmas project at this late date—I should have spoken to her weeks ago! I'll just have my three children decorate them. Let's see, that would come to one hundred bags apiece, with the youngest still in diapers. Hmm … what about inviting all of their friends over for an afternoon of drawing? Yes! We could make it into a neighborhood party—maybe throw in a little caroling as well! Well, now that that's settled, I better focus on getting the bags filled through donations.

My enthusiasm must be contagious because the local businesses are very generous. I now have tons of little gifts, and the hospital kindly donated white bags for the children to decorate.

Yikes—the party is tomorrow! Luckily someone has taken over the dessert portion of this event, and it sounds very well organized. Santa is all lined up as well, and I have hundreds of candy canes that have been donated—probably enough for every child in town. I still haven't figured out when to tackle the bags. The kids are tired, and the house looks like a bomb went off. It will take thirty minutes just to clear the table so that we can start decorating the bags. Too late to call their friends, unfortunately.

Dinner is over, and it's already 8:00 pm. My husband is telling me in a strained voice that it's too late to start such a large project with the kids. No problem. I'll just do it myself after the kids go to bed. But wait, what about the report that was supposed to be finished by tomorrow? I have to write that while I'm still alert. I can always decorate the bags later.

The report took a lot longer than I anticipated, but I'm really happy with the final product. I've read it over six or eight times and made minor changes in wording so now it flows seamlessly. I tried to decorate a bag; but I'm realizing that my artistic talents have not improved since kindergarten, and the bags aren't turning out at all like I had envisioned. My rendition of a decorated Christmas tree looks more like a menacing primeval creature with an unfortunate skin condition. There is no way that I can complete this stupid project. What was I thinking? Tomorrow is a full day at work, so an all-nighter is out of the question. We'll just have to settle for plain white bags. The kids will be thrilled with what's inside!

Back from work now—later than I thought—rummaging through the basement for a box to throw the bags into. The kids aren't bathed yet, but a washcloth should do the trick. Using the kitchen sink as a makeshift bathtub while cooking grilled cheese and giving last-minute instructions to the teenager who has arrived to watch my youngest, we are able to leave the house with seconds to spare. Calling out words of encouragement as my two oldest dash to their classrooms, I rush into the cafeteria prior to the concert, the large box of bags banging wildly against my torso. The other moms, dressed in cute holiday outfits, have already set up a beautiful display of homemade Christmas cookies. I start lining up the bags on a brown laminated lunch table. It's not easy to organize three hundred white bags in a fresh and creative manner, particularly when I forgot to plan for any table decorations. I try to place them randomly, and the table looks like a lost and found for rejected lunch bags. I place them in straight lines, and the bags suddenly look suspiciously like ones you would be given to transport a urine sample to your next OB/GYN appointment.

Gotta run—the concert is starting! Despite the frenetic pace of the past hour, I'm caught up in the magic of childhood as I watch class after class march up on stage, waving to their parents while smiling broadly, elbowing the students next to them, and giggling mid-song. Some stare off into the crowd, seeming to have forgotten that they are supposed to be singing, while others sing out with great gusto, appearing as though this very moment is the highlight of their young lives.

And it's over. I rush back to the cafeteria before the crowd gets there. Here comes Santa! Hey, you look fantastic! Sure, I'll give you a cue when to come out and surprise the kids. The bathroom in the basement? Great idea!

Would you look at the wave of people coming through the door! The room is filling up so quickly. There must be five hundred people in this room! But why is no one picking up a bag? I bet they don't realize that the bags are for the kids. I forgot to make some kind of sign. I'll just head over there and encourage kids to pick them up and look inside. Hmmm … their reaction is less than inspiring. Their eyes are glued to the cookie table, which is beautifully decorated and arranged. The parents look sympathetically in my direction but hurry over to get a cookie themselves.

Thank God, the crowd is starting to thin out. It was so overwhelming; I can't remember talking to a single parent. I hope at least I looked friendly. Glad to see that all the cookies haven't been eaten yet; I'm suddenly famished! Oh good, here comes my wonderful husband, still dressed in his work attire, with the kids in tow. The kids race over to eat the last of the cookies while my husband pitches in to help clean up. The cafeteria has emptied out as quickly as it filled up; only my family and the clean-up crew remains. A member of the clean-up crew is saying, "Wow, it was so busy there for a while, I didn't even notice when Santa came out with the candy canes …"

Oh God. No … no … no … It is NOT possible that he is still in the bathroom. I'm sure I just missed him as well. But on the outside chance, let me go down there and peek in. That way I won't lay awake tonight, wracking my brain, trying to remember Santa's entrance. My husband, with a look that bodes poorly, says that he is going to take the kids home and relieve the babysitter, and while attempting to stifle increasing symptoms of panic, I take off at a fast clip, realizing for the first time that I have no idea where the basement bathroom is even located.

The school kitchen is dark and cavernous. I find my way through, enter a narrow, dimly lit hallway, and see the stairs that descend into the basement. Creeping along, holding my breath, I try to convince myself that Santa will not be in the bathroom when I open the door. I see a shadow through an iced bathroom window. I'm feeling lightheaded and a little nauseous. I open the door, and there he is, a big smile of anticipation on his face. "Are they ready?"

Luckily, this Santa was a particularly kind man, with a sense of humor to boot. He said that he had heard things quieting down upstairs and figured that I had all of the children sitting quietly on the floor, awaiting his entrance. I had to explain, while apologizing profusely, that everyone except the clean-up crew had already left the building.

Rather than becoming miffed, Santa was wonderful and generous in spirit, and offered to come back the next day and go from classroom to classroom, handing out candy canes. I heard later that he was a great hit. I also found out that the "Santa Story" had gone through the school like wildfire, and the teachers all thought that it was hysterically funny. I relayed the story to my parents over Christmas dinner, and my mother had tears of laughter streaming down her face.

Although I could certainly see the humor in the story, I was still stuck with the reality that I had forgotten Santa in the bathroom! So I had to make an action plan to get past it. I made a solemn vow that it would serve as a "learning experience," that I would analyze the situation, think about what I could do differently the next time, and make some changes in my life.

The Santa fiasco took place over fifteen years ago, and since that time a lot of significant changes have indeed taken place. My son was diagnosed with AD/HD, and I was subsequently diagnosed and treated for the disorder as well. Once I was able to focus for extended periods of time, I began to read voraciously on the topic of Attention Deficit/Hyperactivity Disorder. I attended numerous conferences on the subject and decided to focus my practice exclusively on evaluating AD/HD children and adults. As I heard story after story from parents of AD/HD children and from AD/HD adults themselves, I realized that the entire Christmas party, from the beginning planning stages to the sleepless post-party night, consisted of a series of common mistakes that plague AD/HD adults.

It's hard to explain what it's like to discover at the age of thirty-six that you have been struggling with a lifelong disorder. Don't get me wrong—I was very cognizant of the fact that I had always been impulsive, disorganized, forgetful, and inattentive, and I only needed to look at my school report cards for confirmation from each and every one of my teachers. However, not knowing that these were symptoms of a disorder, I had developed numerous theories as to why I did these things, and my theories were for the most part quite self-condemning. I impulsively interrupted others because I was the third child in a sibship of four, and this was my way of demanding attention. Yet I wondered if I would ever be able to move beyond my birth order and behave in a more mature manner. I was unable to concentrate in elementary school because I wasn't one of the "smart kids," and in high school I was more focused on social activities than academics. When I was unable to focus in college, despite a strong desire to do so, I decided that I was suffering from an extended existential crisis, and until I was able to figure out the meaning of life, I would never be able to focus on my textbooks. (To make matters worse, I kept forgetting the term *existential* and would spend valuable study time trying to recall the name of the crisis that I was experiencing.)

Discovering that inattention, impulsivity, and internal restlessness were symptoms of a disorder was a life-altering experience for me. I was still responsible for addressing these behavioral problems; but rather than focusing my energy on belittling myself, I could problem solve and try to determine more effective ways of coping with these symptoms.

Over time, I began to appreciate the value of humor because, despite my knowledge of this disorder and despite my attempts to compensate, I still find myself grappling with AD/HD issues on a daily basis. When you tear your home apart looking for your glasses, only to discover that they are perched atop your head, you have a choice of how to respond. You can berate yourself, feel sorry for yourself, or laugh at the crazy world of the AD/HD adult. I choose to laugh.

Now when I evaluate adults with AD/HD, they invariably state at the end of the morning session: "You know, I was really nervous about coming in, but I learned so much today, and I actually enjoyed myself." I also realize that there are many others out there who are mentally berating themselves, wondering why they continue to make the same mistakes day after day, and asking themselves, "Are you *ever* going to grow up?"

With this in mind, I take on yet another project—using humor to explore the many issues that impact AD/HD adults on a daily basis. Although I recognize that there are serious implications for anyone having this disorder, I also believe that it's never a good idea to take oneself too seriously. Humor unites the AD/HD population and reminds us that we are all in the same boat—even though half the time we cannot remember where we put the oars.

I dedicate this venture to the wonderful parent who, dressed as Santa, waited in a small, overheated basement bathroom for over an hour for a cue that never came. Despite that, this person was so generous in spirit that he came back the next day, dressed once again in full regalia, and handed out a candy cane to each and every child.

Chapter 2

The Elusive Concept of Time

There are many excellent books on Attention Deficit/Hyperactivity Disorder that provide detailed and systematic coverage of central issues, including the history of AD/HD, current diagnostic criteria, the evaluation process, treatment issues, and thoughtful recommendations. This is not one of those books.

Although I recognize as a psychologist the importance of defining this disorder in both historical and scientific terms, as an AD/HD adult I am limited in my writing by my low threshold for boredom and an intolerance of review. So this book will focus on specific issues that I have found to be particularly relevant in the day-to-day functioning of AD/HD adults.

I may err on the side of being too descriptive in my writing, while providing fewer recommendations than is typical of self-help books. I have tried to limit my recommendations to what I have found to be truly helpful for a wide variety of AD/HD adults. Some of what I say will hit home for most AD/HD adults, but no one will agree with everything that is written here. That's the nature of AD/HD.

You will probably notice that every chapter has a somewhat different style and that I drift off on tangents from time to time and insert questionable humor into my writing. Sorry. Although I tried my hardest to create consistency from one chapter to the next, I found the entire process exceedingly dull. My guess is that other AD/HD adults will appreciate the variety and will be less likely to drift off to other thoughts as well. In addition, I promise not to make fun of anything that I don't do myself on a regular basis. Fair enough?

Of the major issues that impact AD/HDers on a daily basis, time management ranks right up at the top of the list. So let's start with the elusive concept of time.

As AD/HD adults, we *know* that there are only twenty-four hours to each day, and that each hour consists of sixty minutes. And by the time we reach our adult years, one would *assume* that we could estimate the passage of time with reasonable accuracy, right? Wrong! In the AD/HD world, an hour can pass by in a millisecond when someone is engrossed in a particularly enjoyable or stimulating activity, and three minutes can feel like an eternity when that person is in a state of forced captivity. Moreover, days and weeks mysteriously disappear, and AD/HD adults are perpetually astonished by the fact that November suddenly turns into December, just when we are getting used to the idea that it is no longer summer.

Time is an incredibly elusive concept in the AD/HD world, one that continually amazes those of us who lose track of it so easily. Unfortunately, this AD/HD trait is one that continually irritates those around us who do not find the passage of time to be such a difficult concept to master.

Let me give you an example. You tell your spouse that you are going to an office supply store for copy paper and that you will be back "in a sec." And that is the plan. You will zip to the store (no traffic, traffic lights, or checkout lines are brought into the equation at this point), and then you will zip back home, jauntily entering the house to a chorus of "Why Mom! You're back already?" But what *really* happens is this: If you are lucky, you will make it into the office supply store without running into someone you know, and locate the copy paper aisle without too much trouble. You'll suddenly remember that the copy paper aisle takes up the length of an entire city block when you are faced with thirty choices of copy paper. Some is on sale; some is on sale only if you buy three or more reams; some is made from recycled paper; some is exclusively for laser printers, and on and on. You finally make your selection based on a form of logic that has already eluded you, and on your way to the checkout counter you happen to pass by the personal planner aisle. Anyone with AD/HD knows the incredible pull that the personal planner aisle has on an AD/HDers psyche. Why, there may be a solution to our disorganization only a few steps away!

While in the process of trying to determine whether daily or weekly planners are more effective and whether a zippered case would serve as the kiss of death to any organizational system that you might develop, your cell phone rings, and your spouse, who is inexplicably furious, reminds you that your daughter's Girl Scout meeting starts in fifteen minutes. She cannot find her outfit in the heap of dirty laundry, and you have the only working car in the family.

What is most amazing is that when double-checking your watch, being certain that your spouse is overreacting once again, you realize that you have been gone from home for over an hour! So, how in the world did you lose track of that much time?

I have put a lot of thought into this issue, given the fact that time loss is a recurrent problem for me. For a while, I favored the idea that I was repeatedly being abducted by aliens, a hypothesis that I still fall back on from time to time. Although this may sound a tad far-fetched to the uninitiated, it's exactly what it feels like when you are jolted out of a state of reverie, only to discover that you once again have lost track of a large chunk of time. I offered this particular explanation to my husband so many times while the kids were growing up that, coupled with my strange behavior, they began to wonder if I indeed *was* an alien. In fact, when my youngest daughter first heard the term *legal alien* on a news program, she turned and looked at me with newfound respect.

Although my alien abduction theory is one that resonates most closely with my experience of time loss, when I seriously review the events that lead up to these time warps, it usually boils down to the fact that I become distracted and then consumed by other activities or thoughts (for example, the leather-bound planner *looks* the best, but it won't look so hot when I find it underneath the car seat next month along with a couple of soggy pretzels and a half-eaten candy bar). Plus, if I were so lucky as to be abducted by aliens, it would only happen once, and the visit would end abruptly when they realized that they had abducted a defective model.

Losing track of time appears to occur when the AD/HD individual is intensely involved in something. Hallowell and Ratey (1994) argue that the term *attention deficit* is in fact a misnomer and that *attention inconsistency* would be a more accurate term.[2] When an AD/HDer is caught up in a particularly interesting activity, he or she often "over-focuses" to the point of tuning out his or her environment and losing track of time. This can be a source of much confusion for family members who are trying to make sense of the AD/HDer's behavior. Many parents have told me that there is no way that their children can have AD/HD, because they can become so absorbed in activities that they enjoy. Many spouses of AD/HD adults have come to the erroneous conclusion that they are not valued or that they play second fiddle in the worlds of their inattentive partners, who can be absorbed for hours in projects but will drift off in conversation.

Losing track of large chunks of time is only one aspect of time perception problems for AD/HD adults. On the other end of the spectrum, time can go by at an agonizingly slow pace at other points of your day. Being forced, for example, to wait for the car in front of you to make a left turn can feel like waiting for an eternity, during which time you add to your children's fund of words that they should never say in front of their friends or their teachers. I have posed the following question to many AD/HD adults in my practice: If you had a choice to a) wait an indefinite length of time to make a left turn across traffic or b) make a right turn and drive three miles out of your way to get to your destination, which would you prefer? Invariably the AD/HD adult will look at me as if I were daft and say, "Why, the second choice, of course!" Waiting is *not* something that AD/HD people do by choice.

This intense aversion to waiting, I believe, is one reason why AD/HD adults are so often late for appointments. Clearly, they do not want to arrive five minutes prior to their scheduled appointment time and be forced to sit in a waiting room reading outdated magazine articles. Therefore, the plan is always to get there right on time. Unfortunately, arriving "right on time" requires a proficiency in time estimation—a skill that is oddly lacking in the AD/HD population.

What do non-AD/HDers do when they have only five minutes before they have to leave the house for an appointment? I have no idea, actually, but my guess is that it does not involve a frenzy of activity that would parallel the intensity of an Olympic event. For an AD/HD adult, however, the words "five minutes before we have to leave" releases a burst of adrenaline whose expression cannot be denied.

First, have you ever noticed that although your house may have been trashed for the past twenty-four hours, five minutes before you are supposed to leave the house for an appointment, you are suddenly overwhelmed with the urge to put things back in their proper places? It also seems that the longer you are planning to be away, the cleaner your house has to be before you can walk out the door. I can't count the number of planes we have almost missed because of this last-minute (but never planned for) cleaning craze that comes over me. The last time this happened, I was certain that my husband would not speak to me for the entire "romantic weekend" that we were away.

Next, without question, AD/HDers are most productive when there is a clear and imminent deadline looming before them, and the desire to take advantage of this surge of productivity is overwhelming. "Let me just toss these dishes in the dishwasher, quickly make that eye appointment, and then throw in a load of laundry so that my son's choir uniform is ready for tonight's concert." Due to our optimistic natures, we are certain that we can do all of this in the five minutes before we absolutely, positively must leave the house.

Furthermore, as mentioned earlier, when planning to make an appointment across town, traffic and available parking spaces never seem to enter into the equation. Nor do we seem to remember that most people abide by the speed limit when driving, a practice that drives many AD/HDers mad with frustration, particularly when they have only five minutes to get to their destinations. Although I have been guilty of cursing the driver in front of me for having the audacity to drive the posted speed limit, I am simultaneously aware of the horrific statistics associated with AD/HD and driving.[3]

If AD/HD adults are chronically late for appointments, why is it that we do not learn from experience? Scholarly articles and books have consistently noted that individuals with AD/HD do not learn from experience to the same degree as our non-AD/HD counterparts, and it has been hypothesized that we do not benefit from the feedback that we receive from our environment[4] and do not inhibit our initial reaction ("Go for it!") in order to plan effectively for the future.[5]

Although these well-researched and thoughtful theories may bear validity, I would like to offer an alternative explanation: that AD/HD individuals are outrageously (and often unjustifiably) optimistic by nature. Thus, although I realize that prior experience has *suggested* that I cannot make it across town in under twenty minutes, at the moment that I am making my plans, I am brimming with a sense of wellbeing and certitude that I can indeed defy all odds and make the trip in eighteen minutes flat. (This personal theory of optimism provides clear support for the scholarly treatises mentioned above.)

Now, I promised at the beginning of this book that I would not make excuses for AD/HD traits. Being late can be very annoying for those who assume that events should start promptly. So how do you work around this?

- Set your watch alarm to go off ten minutes before you have to leave the house. When it goes off, stop whatever you are doing *immediately* and get going! Do not, under any circumstances, finish the solitaire game that you are playing, and if the phone rings, let the caller know that you *cannot* talk. I once missed an important meeting that I had planned my entire afternoon around because I answered the phone and got caught up in conversation. ("She did *what*? When did *this* happen?") And believe it or not, I did not think of the meeting again until hours later when something jarred my memory.
- Plan to arrive ten minutes early. In theory, this will allow you to drive leisurely (leisurely *adj*: without haste) to your appointment and provide you the opportunity to relax and regroup. Then, when everything goes wrong, as it invariably does, you will end up arriving at your appointment right on time. Think about it. How many times have you said: "I *would* have been on time if it hadn't been for ..." Why not assume that these things will indeed pop up and *plan* for them? You cannot, however, purposely add another last-minute activity to your list, knowing that you have allowed for wiggle room in your schedule. That, unfortunately, defeats the purpose. If you somehow manage to arrive before your appointment time, bring a good novel or a book of puzzles so that you are not driven mad by the wait. Cleaning out your purse or wallet will also do in a pinch.
- Keep your car keys in the same spot. How many events have you been late for because at the last minute you cannot locate your keys?
- Put items that you need to bring with you out on the counter the night before so that when you wake up the next morning in a befuddled fog, everything will be in one place. This can include the book that you may need to stave off boredom on the outside chance that you arrive early for an appointment. For those of you who are wondering "What book is she talking

about?", it's time to take a break. We'll discuss the problem of reading retention in a later chapter.

- Don't wait until the last minute to get dressed. This will help avoid that moment of panic (and the inevitable delay) when you realize that you do not have any clean underwear and that your hair is protruding at odd angles from your scalp.
- When you think of something you need to do at the last minute, *just say no*! This apparently worked for Nancy Reagan, and in theory it should work for AD/HD adults as well.

Chapter 3

Organization and the Best Laid Plans

A few years ago, after I entertained my sister during a weeklong stay, she sent a couple of books to me on "organizing your home and life." Mind you, the timing of this gift did not go unnoticed. Luckily, I decided to glance over the introductory pages as a gesture of courtesy to my sister who, I thought with righteous indignation, knew nothing about courtesy herself. I did not anticipate that, as I opened the first book and began to read reluctantly, it would describe a life the likes of which I had yet to fathom. It was akin to the moment when the hero of *The Truman Show* realized that there was a huge world out there whose existence had heretofore been hidden from him.

I'm somewhat embarrassed to admit that basic concepts of organization were true revelations to me. One author noted, for example, that kitchen cupboards should be organized in such a manner that items that are used on a daily basis are placed within arms reach, while seasonal items are put away in storage and retrieved only as the season approaches. While this may be common sense to those who are not organizationally impaired, I was thunderstruck by the notion that I did not have to push aside Christmas coffee mugs each morning in search of one that was seasonally appropriate the other eleven months of the year.

After reading the first few chapters, I could not contain my excitement any longer and set about to reorganize the house. My plan was to start in the kitchen and to move from room to room until I lived in a model home of organization and efficiency. The enthusiasm that I carried into this project was truly awe-inspiring, and I can still remember the grand visions that I entertained of a sparkling home where there was a place for everything and everything was in its place. It all seemed so very easy—if only I had been aware of the organizational literature a little earlier in my life!

Since I need to remain honest in these "memoirs," I have to admit that my organizational efforts never made it past the kitchen. You see, as is typical of AD/HD adults, as I became more and more involved in my organizing project, I began to ignore all other aspects of my life, such as my work responsibilities and my children's schedules. (I wonder if it was at this point that I was "fired" by my dentist due to the large number of missed appointments.)

With hindsight, I realize that in my excitement over this novel concept called organization, I moved into a state of hyperfocus, a frame of mind that AD/HDers experience when particularly interested in or enthusiastic about a task or subject matter. Hyperfocus is characterized by an intense, single-minded focus that often obliterates any other unrelated thought, such as having to pick up your children from school or needing to take dinner out of the oven. If made available in pill form, hyperfocus would be classified as a highly addictive, euphoria-inducing drug for AD/HDers and would quickly be taken off the market by the FDA for being "too much fun." The capacity to hyperfocus is what makes highly successful AD/HDers highly successful, and it has been speculated that during periods of hyperfocus, AD/HDers can focus better than the average person. Hyperfocus, like all other really fun things, unfortunately, has its drawbacks, because during these periods of intense focus, all other responsibilities are pushed aside,[6] which brings us back to the story of my failed attempt at a Martha Stewart lifestyle.

In addition to losing track of time and children while organizing my kitchen, I also lost track of my general cleaning plan and began to focus on smaller and smaller details. It suddenly became tremendously important, for example, to touch up the small rust spots in the back corners of my forty-year-old metal kitchen cabinets, although every other room in the house had reached a state where a Protective Service referral would have been in order. At some point, after realizing that I was dreadfully behind at work and that my children had taken up residence with neighbors who still served meals, I called it quits on a project that has hence been referred to in my family as The Kitchen Organizing Fiasco.

The tendency to focus on details while overlooking the larger picture, a common feature of AD/HD, has been a persistent and incredibly exasperating problem throughout my adult life, particularly when housework is involved. If, for example, I am planning a dinner party for eight, rather than focusing on food preparation and cleaning the rooms where we will be entertaining that very evening, I inexplicably find myself spending the majority of the afternoon reorganizing the work bench in the basement or rearranging my daughter's Barbie clothes by color and season.

In *ADD-Friendly Ways to Organize Your Life*, Judith Kohlberg and Dr. Kathleen Nadeau identify this tendency to get lost in the details of an organizational project as slipping into "micro-focus." These authors suggest that going into micro-focus is a means by which AD/HDers shield themselves from feeling overwhelmed by the larger project at hand. This makes a lot of sense to me, and I do indeed feel a tremendous sense of peace while cleaning lint from the back panel of my dryer prior to a fancy dinner party that I am hosting. Yet I cannot help but wonder why I do not micro-focus on the food that I should be preparing or on the correct pronunciation of our guests' last names.

When talking to AD/HD adults, another organizational issue that comes up again and again is the problem with piles—piles of school papers, piles of mail, piles of articles that you were planning to read, piles of little yellow sticky notes with important reminders. Actually, AD/HDers don't have a problem with piles—in fact we really like our piles. Yet there is always this nagging feeling that June Cleaver in "Leave it to Beaver" or Margaret Anderson in "Father Knows Best" never had piles of papers covering every horizontal surface in their homes. Any adult with AD/HD, however, knows the true value of piles—they are vertical arrangements of reminders of things that we need to do. If these piles are systematically put away, as suggested in most organizational handbooks, these responsibilities will be forgotten completely.

In another one of my organizational crazes, I decided to tackle my personal papers. As is the case with many AD/HDers, while my work files were arranged with an obsessive attention to detail, my home files were in complete and total disarray. In fact, prior to being introduced to the organizational literature, it never occurred to me to arrange my personal papers in an orderly manner, and although I would spend an entire afternoon trying to locate my daughter's birth certificate so that she could be enrolled in kindergarten, I assumed that everyone went through this same process.

When, however, I learned that piles of unread papers were organizational no-nos, I cheerfully decided to adopt a three-pile method that would eliminate all paper clutter and allow me to have any specific document at my fingertips at a moment's notice. Over the course of a week or two, I went through my most current piles and divided them into three groups: Group A consisted of those papers that could be thrown away; Group B was reserved for papers that needed to be filed and saved; and Group C was for papers that needed to be reviewed (but not necessarily saved).

Before long my desk and counter tops were cleared, and everything was either thrown out or put away in file folders labeled: "To File" or "To Review." I was so very pleased with my mastery of organizational techniques that I shared my newfound knowledge with a client whom I was evaluating for AD/HD. "Hmmm," she replied, "and when do you take the time to review and file the papers?" I stared at her, dumbstruck and momentarily speechless, realizing for the first time that I hadn't even thought about this logical next step. And I was once again reminded of the adage that perpetuates the piling system of AD/HDers: "Out of sight, out of mind."

I have come to the conclusion that I am a binge organizer, although there is far too little purging that takes place. Although I do not wish to appear pessimistic in outlook, I have also come to the conclusion that due to the very nature of AD/HD, consistent adherence to *any* organizational system is an unreasonable expectation. Individuals with AD/HD crave stimulation, and when in a setting where this need for stimulation is undernourished, AD/HDers will unconsciously take matters into their own hands and create the stimulation that they desire.

Let's apply this theory to an organizational scheme. You go to an office supply store and buy all of the necessary accoutrements for a dynamite organizational system. You may decide on color-coded folders for your papers or an accordion-style organizer with monthly pockets for your bills. You may spend an entire weekend organizing all of your current papers. (Less current papers are in a box somewhere in the basement or perhaps the attic.) This system is fresh and exciting, and it initially is quite stimulating to maintain. But over time (perhaps a week or even a month), the system loses its appeal. What's interesting is that AD/HD adults do not appear to be consciously aware of their waning interest in their most recent organizational scheme—rather, they just seem to completely put it out of their minds and are almost startled when the memory of this organizational system resurfaces, like the face of a distant relative that they haven't thought of in years.

In *Driven to Distraction,* Hallowell and Ratey note that individuals with AD/HD have an intolerance for boredom, and they go on to state: "Actually the person with ADD seldom feels bored. This is because the millisecond he senses boredom, he swings into action and finds something new; he changes the channel."[7] This would help to explain how an organizational system can be forgotten so completely. The Organizational Channel becomes dull and repetitive, so the AD/HD individual begins channel surfing until he or she finds one that holds his or her attention, at least for the moment.

When I have tried to retrace the steps of my organizational demise, most often it is due to the fact that I became involved in a project of greater interest. Maybe it was the purchase of an electric guitar and the ensuing belief that I would soon be playing lovely ballads while sitting cross-legged on the floor, surrounded by burning incense. Perhaps it was the start of an exercise craze when I became determined to swim three-quarters of a mile per day until my body took on the buffed appearance of an eighteen-year-old swimsuit model. Or maybe it was another organizational project that caught my fancy, such as creating a scrapbook for each of my four children, which entailed going through boxes and boxes of school papers and drawings that dated back to preschool. Each of these fleeting fancies have indeed occurred. In fact they have all taken place within the past three months!

Thus, I have to make a politically (or psychologically) incorrect confession. The idea of having a completely organized life sounds *to me* like a death sentence. I honestly don't care if I handle a piece of paper more than once (a big no-no in the organizational literature), and frankly it gives me the heebie-jeebies to even think about functioning at this level of micro-management. It's not that I am ignoring the importance of organization—that would be truly foolhardy in the AD/HD world. In fact, I am quite zealous in my adherence to the overriding organizational principle that I live by, which is *to avoid falling into a state of complete chaos.*

Lest the reader makes the faulty assumption that I am being facetious in what is a serious matter, let me explain the logic behind my organizational goal. Through personal experience, I have found that when I fall sufficiently behind in meeting my responsibilities, rather than becoming motivated to pull it together, the exact opposite occurs—I enter into a state of psychological paralysis.[8] Although I am aware of all that needs to be done and feel a growing sense of panic that accompanies deadlines that have been ignored, I am unable to make any headway in terms of planning how to meet my responsibilities. Rather, I enter into a stupefied state in which I am only capable of playing endless games of solitaire. I have spoken to countless AD/HD adults who describe the "swimming" sensation that takes place in their minds as they try to tackle what feels like an overwhelming number of responsibilities. This feeling of helplessness is truly frightening, so frightening, in fact, that I have developed an entire system of warning signals to indicate when I'm getting dangerously close to the abyss.

A low-level alert sounds for me when I notice that my to-do list has morphed into an accumulation of yellow sticky notes that are placed haphazardly across the face of my computer monitor. Other signals that indicate the beginning of an organizational decline are when I find my planner in various places around the house, instead of in my purse where it belongs, and when I realize for the third evening in a row that calling to schedule a dentist appointment must take place between the hours of 8:00 am and 5:00 pm.

A medium-level alert signal goes off when sticky notes begin to accumulate on the bathroom mirror, the kitchen cupboards, and on the glass panes of the back door. Additional alert signals sound when, while looking for my misplaced cell phone, I find my organizer stuck between the seats of the car. Realizing while getting my hair styled that I forgot to arrange to have the kids picked up from school also falls into this mid-level category.

A high-level alert signal is activated when the sticky notes begin to fall behind my desk, and when I start to find them on the floor of the car, with shoe prints and dirt marks obliterating key words, when I sleep through my alarm and miss the parent-teacher conference that was scheduled for 11:00 am, and when I realize that I haven't seen—or even thought about—my organizer in days. I try not to let my life deteriorate to this point, but when it does, I leap into high gear and begin reinstituting my basic organizational structure, knowing that psychological paralysis is the next stage in my organizational decline.

And I can honestly say that I cannot remember the last time I experienced this level of chaos in my life. (Although given the current state of my memory, that's really not saying much, is it?) Sure, I receive low-level alerts quite regularly, but it's easy to regroup at this point. When there is a lot going on in my life, I will begin to notice moderately high alert signals, and then I know I need an afternoon to pull it together. But with this system in place, I am confident that my enjoyment of spontaneity will not evolve into a life of chaos. For me this is organizational success.

Chapter 4

The Art of Conversation

If Communication 101: The Art of Conversation were to be offered at local community colleges, the classrooms would be jam-packed with AD/HD adults who have berated themselves for years over their conversational faux pas. Of course, one would need really dynamic instructors or else the classes would quickly deteriorate into total mayhem as class members interrupted each other, went off on seemingly unrelated tangents, and argued incessantly over the meaning of the word *art*.

Why do AD/HD adults struggle so much with the art of conversation? I believe that there are many, many reasons, which is why this topic gets its own chapter. These would include the tendency to lose focus, short-term memory deficits, the overwhelming desire to interrupt, and the confusing habit of jumping from point A to point Z, while assuming that your listener "gets" the connection. Other frequently mentioned communication problems include difficulty keeping up with fast-paced banter, difficulty organizing one's thoughts, and problems with word retrieval—that is, finding the right words, or any words for that matter, to express oneself.

The tendency to drift off in conversation is a frequently cited problem of AD/HD adults and their frustrated partners. Drifting off does not necessarily imply that the speaker is deadly boring, and most frequently the AD/HD adult is unaware that he or she has "left the building." If AD/HD individuals have an issue that is consuming them, although they may *intend* to focus on the conversation, they often find themselves repeatedly sidetracked by competing concerns. The issue that may be consuming the AD/HD adult does not have to be a critical one, such as: "My landlord is going to evict me if this check bounces" or "Maybe the pink hue on my home pregnancy test was due to the lighting in the bathroom." Rather, the AD/HDer may be incessantly reviewing a comment that was made to him or her in a previous conversation and wondering if the comment was intended to be as insulting as it sounded.

It's quite embarrassing to suddenly realize that there is a pause in the conversation and the speaker is staring at you in anticipation, awaiting your response. And our tendency to drift off is no doubt a source of great frustration to our conversational partners, unless they themselves have AD/HD, in which case they may have drifted off to other thoughts as well. This issue was mentioned to me recently by an AD/HD college student who had gone through several roommates over the course of the year, and she acknowledged that her request for her roommates to "start all over" in conversation was never well received.

Another situation where AD/HDers typically lose focus is when the speaker is repeating something that he or she has already said—perhaps several times in the past. The process of listening to overlearned material provides no stimulation for the AD/HD brain, and it will automatically seek out something of greater interest value or shut down in defeat. This may be why many AD/HD adults dislike cocktail parties and the mode of conversation that dominates these events. After repeating the standard cocktail party mantra ten or twelve times over the course of an hour, the AD/HD adult is at risk for developing CPS, Cocktail Party Stupor, a mental state characterized by a five- to ten-word vocabulary, disjointed verbalizations that do not contain both a noun and a verb, as well as responses that are only vaguely related to the topics at hand. I should mention that although Cocktail Party Stupor can be magnified by alcohol intake, it cannot be avoided by remaining sober. You see, CPS is not caused by alcohol consumption, rather it reflects sorely understimulated frontal lobes.

Speakers who talk slowly or those who do not come up for air for extended periods of time will also lose their AD/HD listeners, that is, those AD/HD listeners who have not already bolted from the room, screaming in psychic pain. This brings up an issue that is near and dear to me. Why is it that children are chided from early on when they interrupt in conversation, and adults who interrupt are considered to be social pariahs, yet those who drone on incessantly are never corrected? I think there should be some sort of parity that begins in kindergarten. Just as a teacher will tell a child, "Johnny, it is not polite to interrupt," he or she should also say with equal frequency: "Fred, your droning, tedious description is causing great discomfort for your more lively classmates!"

Short-term memory deficits can also wreak havoc on the AD/HDer's ability to follow a conversation, and although they may stay focused on what is currently being discussed, everything that has been said prior to that point may have already been forgotten. In our household, my children find great humor in the fact that I happily bounce along in conversation like an overactive golden retriever on a walk through the park. Sometimes I race off to chase a squirrel (bringing up tangential issues that serve more to distract than to promote the conversation), but I cheerfully rejoin them when cued. However, if they happen to go back to a previous topic, perhaps one that was discussed only moments before, I will often have no idea what they are talking about. Below would be a typical mother-daughter conversation in our household:

Daughter:	Mom, can Colleen spend the night tomorrow?
Mother:	Why? What's going on?
Daughter:	Her parents are going to be out of town, and she's been pretty upset lately; so I said that I'd ask you if she could come over and hang out.
Mother:	Why is she upset?
Daughter:	Well, her boyfriend is being a jerk, at least that's what she says, although I haven't heard the whole story yet.
Mother:	You mean Ken?
Daughter:	Yeah.
Mother:	Hmmm, I don't know what to think about him. Isn't he the one who wouldn't take her to prom?
Daughter:	That was last year, and they weren't dating then, so can she?
Mother:	Can who?
Daughter:	Colleen!
Mother:	What?

Luckily my children have the patience of saints, and they find their dotty old mother rather amusing. The inability to keep track of topics throughout a conversation is more of a problem, however, when talking to someone who is unaware of the fact that your short-term memory rivals that of a fruit fly. I can't tell you the number of times that I have received a phone call that starts out with a specific request ("Would you be willing to lead the Girl Scout troop on Saturday?") and then moves on to various other topics, and by the time I have hung up the phone, the fact that I have agreed to lead the Girl Scout troop has completely and totally left my mind. When talking to good friends, I typically ask them to remind me at the end of the conversation why they called in the first place, and they do so with good humor. This is not the best tactic to use, however, when talking to your child's teacher, and for these conversations, it's good to have a pen and sticky pad on hand.

This brings me to the next conversational blunder of AD/HD adults—the granddaddy of them all—the tendency to interrupt. Let me preface this section by stating that one of the most enjoyable aspects of talking to AD/HD adults for me *is* their tendency to interrupt, as well as their affable acceptance of being interrupted in return. Yes, I realize that the habit of interrupting is often infuriating to non-AD/HD individuals, who view it as rude, insensitive, and disrespectful. Interrupting in the AD/HD world, however, is another way of saying: "Yep—gotcha, and let me add this food for thought." You can discuss twice as many ideas by not insisting on finishing every sentence! It is truly amazing how two AD/HD individuals can get on the same wavelength and know on some psychic level what the other person is about to say.

Unfortunately, when the founders of Conversation Etiquette convened to determine the rules and regulations of their field, the AD/HD contingent was not invited to participate. Or perhaps they were, but they misplaced their invitations and forgot to RSVP until it was too late. Whatever the particular circumstances were, it was determined by the non-AD/HD majority that interrupting was not to be tolerated in anyone older than the age of three, unless there was a *dire* emergency. (The definition of *dire emergency* was no doubt spelled out in painful detail, and therefore has never been read in its entirety by anyone with attentional deficits.)

In defense of those of us who just can't seem to master the "wait until they're finished" rule, let me fill the reader in on the AD/HD perspective. One reason that AD/HDers interrupt is because they incorrectly assume that their conversation partner has already finished speaking, or at least he or she has *covered the essence* of what he or she wanted to say. Under these circumstances, AD/HDers are actually quite surprised to discover that they *have* indeed interrupted. Hallowell and Ratey note that AD/HDers "love bottom lines"[9] and prefer to "cut to the chase" in conversation. Having to listen to an unabridged version of almost any story can be quite painful for the restless AD/HD adult.

Another reason that AD/HD individuals interrupt is due to a fear that if they wait until the speaker has finished his or her sentence, they will completely forget what it is they wanted to say. For students in class, I recommend writing down questions or comments, and then waiting for an appropriate moment to present them. This technique also works when talking to someone on the phone. In casual, face-to-face conversations, however, this technique could prove to be a bit awkward: "Excuse me for a moment while I retrieve a pen and pad of paper so that I can be writing down my thoughts while you speak." No matter how you phrase that, it would still go over like a lead balloon, which is unfortunate, because if the particularly polite AD/HDer chooses not to interrupt, he or she will become consumed by the effort that is required to remember what he or she wanted to say and will miss out entirely on the other side of the dialogue.

Sometimes AD/HDers interrupt because the desire to express a thought is so overpowering that it feels like an erupting volcano. Of course, after the statement has been blurted out and an uncomfortable silence ensues, the AD/HDer realizes that he or she has once again behaved like a social misfit, and this provides fodder for the late night self-recrimination sessions that often occur in the AD/HD mind. (It's amazing how well we remember every social blunder that we commit over the course of a day, yet we cannot for the life of us remember to take the overdue videos back to the store.)

Another communication faux pas, monopolizing conversations, can occur when the AD/HD individual is really fired up. Recognizing that others are not as enthralled with your ideas as you are will go a long way toward getting you invited to future get-togethers.

For adults with predominant symptoms of inattention, interrupting and monopolizing conversation are not as much of a problem as the process of keeping up with rapid banter. Many inattentive clients express frustration over their inability to process ideas and organize responses in a rapid enough manner to contribute actively in conversation, and they are left feeling socially inept and frustrated. Difficulty with word retrieval is also common for many adults with AD/HD, both with and without hyperactivity, and this is exacerbated when the individual feels uncomfortable or self-conscious. I am not referring to complex or technical word choices—at times the act of putting together a simple sentence seems next to impossible.

Skipping from A to Z is a problem unless both speakers have AD/HD. What often happens is that while the non-AD/HD person is talking, the AD/HD individual is leaping from point A to B and on to point C in his or her mind, and when the AD/HDer enthusiastically pipes in with point G, he or she often gets a look that is typically reserved for those displaying flagrant signs of psychosis. When talking to another AD/HD individual, these leaps seem perfectly natural, and the acrobatics that occur when two AD/HDers are talking can be quite amusing. An inherent danger of leapfrogging in conversation is when your mind leaps past points B and C before *you* finish verbalizing point A, and then you are accused of stopping in mid-sentence, which is *technically* true although the rest of the sentence, as well as several others, have already been completed in your mind. And if you are actually following this discourse, go immediately to the nearest mental health clinic and ask to be evaluated for AD/HD!

At the beginning of this chapter, I posed the question: "Why do AD/HD adults struggle so much with the art of conversation?" Increasing evidence indicates that the problems of inattention associated with AD/HD are secondary to an impairment in executive functioning.[10] The role of executive functioning in the brain has been likened to the position of CEO in a large company. No, I am not talking about robbing tens of thousands of employees of their hard-earned pensions. Executive functions are management functions of the brain, and they "activate, regulate and integrate a wide variety of other mental functioning."[11] When executive functioning is impaired, a broad range of secondary problems will be exhibited.

Executive dysfunction includes problems with working memory,[12] sustained attention, verbal fluency, and processing speed,[13] and each of these functions clearly impact communication skills. *Working memory* deficits can be seen in the struggles that AD/HDers have when attempting to listen while simultaneously organizing a response. Problems with *sustained attention* in conversation are legendary for AD/HDers, and as mentioned previously in this chapter, many AD/HD adults drift off in conversation. *Verbal fluency* relates to the ability to put together a sentence that includes words other than *umm, hmm, errr*, and *yeah*, and although AD/HDers can talk a blue streak on topics of their own choosing, they experience an exasperating shutdown of cognitive functioning when the conversation suddenly veers to black holes or historical events that are recalled by everyone except those who suffer from AD/HD. Finally, *processing speed* impacts the rate at which AD/HDers can follow a conversation and adeptly interject a response, and this seems to be more of a problem for the inattentive subgroup.

All in all, verbal communication seems to broadcast the core deficits of AD/HD. It's no wonder that AD/HD adults mention problems with communication as a central concern!

What great gems of wisdom can I offer to assist those with conversational impairments? First and foremost, if you find yourself talking to someone who drones on and on in an affected tone of voice, immediately feign illness and run off in search of the nearest exit. Second, unless you are talking to a fellow AD/HDer, interrupting is still a social taboo, and the cool stares that you receive are truly more painful than the internal restlessness that builds until you are sure that you are going to burst a blood vessel. Third, if you are really distracted by another issue, it's good policy to be up front about it and say, "I'm very sorry but I am so distracted right now. But I really do want to hear about your _____. Could we talk about it later?" Finally, with an understanding non-AD/HD friend, you can say, "Remind me to tell you about _____. Now go on with what you were saying!" For obvious reasons, this technique is not recommended when talking to a fellow AD/HDer, since the chances that either one of you will remember what you wanted to say are slim to none.[14]

Chapter 5

The Gift and the Curse of Hyperfocus

After reading through portions of my rough draft, my nine-year-old daughter looked up at me suspiciously and asked, "You *did* get your PhD, didn't you?" The answer to that is "Yes—with flying colors" due to the incredible gift of hyperfocus. After spending more time aggravating my teachers in high school than learning the material, and after perfecting the art of last-minute cramming in college, I discovered a field of study that fascinated me. Over the course of the next four years of graduate training, I immersed myself in the field of clinical psychology and focusing in class was no longer a problem.

A greater concern for me was focusing on any *other* aspect of my life, and it's a testament to my husband's character that he was able to tolerate my single-minded purpose during those early years of marriage. I do remember one occasion during the writing of my dissertation when he asked with frustration, "Why didn't you tell me that I would be marrying an obsessive-compulsive?" At that time I was unaware of the concept of hyperfocus and probably gave the matter only momentary consideration before becoming engrossed once again in my studies.

As mentioned previously, Hallowell and Ratey, leading authors in the field of AD/HD, have noted that the term *attentional deficit* is misleading.[15] If interested in a topic, an individual with AD/HD can focus very well—to the point of tuning out his or her environment and losing track of time. This extreme focus has been referred to as hyperfocus,[16] and when applied to a field of interest, hyperfocus can be a key ingredient to professional success. For those who have not experienced this wonderful high, let me give you a rundown on hyperfocus:

- Hyperfocus occurs when an AD/HDer immerses himself or herself in a topic or activity that is intrinsically motivating and enjoyable.
- During these periods of hyperfocus, there is a clarity of thought and a level of creativity that may arguably make up for the hours of muddled thinking that occur at other points in the AD/HDer's day.
- Hyperfocusing is all encompassing in terms of one's attention and focus, and the sense of well-being that one experiences at such times can be likened to falling in love: you are invested in something larger than yourself, and all is right with the world.[17]
- Because hyperfocus involves total immersion in an area of interest, it is essentially a solitary activity. Even if there are other people in the immediate vicinity, they are tuned out.
- Although hyperfocus cannot be induced on demand, one can clearly create an environment that is conducive to hyperfocusing. Having no direct interruptions is, of course, critical, but while some AD/HDers require a complete absence of distracting stimuli in order to move into a state of hyperfocus, others need a certain level of background noise in order to lose themselves in their work (or play).
- Hyperfocus can occur when engaged in primarily cognitive activities, such as reading, writing, creating, or problem solving. Hyperfocus can also take place when an AD/HDer is taking part in more physical activities, such as exercising, gardening, participating in sporting events, or organizing one's front closet.

Over the past thirteen years, I have evaluated hundreds of adults for AD/HD, and I marvel at the wide range of talents and gifts that these individuals possess. They may be teachers, physicians, judges, lawyers, stay-at-home parents, therapists, contractors, plumbers, painters, landscapers, architects, artists of all kinds, and adults who volunteer their time and energy to a wide variety of causes. These individuals share a spirit, a commitment, and a passion for what they do—and they all describe the state of hyperfocus that they experience when engaged in what is truly meaningful to them.

While the state of hyperfocus is often spoken of in reverent tones within the AD/HD community, the ability to focus to such an extreme has its disadvantages as well, particularly in terms of one's interpersonal relationships. You see, when hyperfocusing, what feels like ten minutes to the AD/HD adult may in fact be two hours or more, resulting in missed appointments, late arrivals, burnt dinners, and a reputation for being inconsistently and exasperatingly unreliable. In addition, given the intensity and the all-encompassing nature of hyperfocus, AD/HDers essentially tune out all other aspects of their environment. They may not register their adolescent's request to "borrow the family car for the evening," their partner's attempts at conversation, or the baby crying in the next room. A few years back, there was a house fire directly across the street from our home, and although the lights of the fire trucks created a strobe effect across the walls of my study and the voices of neighbors could be heard from inside our house, I was so caught up in the writing of a report that I was impervious to the sounds and sights of this drama for the first hour that it was unfolding.

As one can imagine, losing track of large chunks of time while completely tuning out one's surroundings is not the best way to show how much you care for those around you. One particular incident stands out in my mind as a turning point in my early parenting years, which led me to give up many extracurricular activities that encouraged hyperfocus for an extended period of time.

Around the time that I forgot Santa in the bathroom, I was working part-time and parenting three young children. We lived in an old house that had definitely seen better days, and any home improvement project, no matter how limited in its initial scope, ended up being a costly and time-consuming endeavor (a fact that I seemed to forget from one home improvement project to the next.) The front door of this house had a wooden panel that was split from years of exposure to northern Michigan elements, and one day a neighbor of mine suggested that the panel could be replaced with a stained glass window. This neighbor kindly offered to lend me his glass cutting equipment as well as his expertise; and the next thing I knew, a beautiful design had been created by a local stained glass studio, and my study had been transformed into a stained glass workshop. The fact that I had never in my life worked with stained glass did not deter me, nor did it seem unrealistic that my first project would be a three-by-five-foot panel fashioned after an intricate Frank Lloyd Wright design. Knowing my poor time estimation skills, I probably assumed that I could create the glass panel over the course of a long weekend, working only when the children were napping or were in bed for the night.

I have very few memories of those weeks that I immersed myself in this project, sneaking into my office at every conceivable moment, like an addict with an overwhelming craving to cut and place "one more piece." I can remember my neighbor telling me that each piece of glass need not be perfect. I can also remember ignoring his advice and returning to the stained glass store repeatedly for additional glass to replace the pieces whose edges were ever so slightly flawed. (Perhaps another attribute that should be added to the description of hyperfocus is the inability to absorb or even acknowledge alternative perspectives.)

During this time, my children were discouraged from entering the room for fear that they might bump the worktable and dislodge hundreds of pieces of glass that had been painstakingly cut and placed; and I can remember my daughter toddling into the room one evening to say goodnight, and my reaction being one of irritation at being interrupted. (Interrupting an AD/HDer in the midst of hyperfocus does not elicit the best of responses.) I have no memories of my husband during this period of time, although I can imagine that he upped his parenting duties while trying in vain to encourage me to use a modicum of moderation when approaching this newfound passion.

I clearly recall that the final project was truly amazing—so well crafted that the owner of the stained glass studio accused my neighbor of doing it himself and creating competition for her business. It was so in keeping with the style of the house that subsequent owners researched the design on the Internet, assuming that it was an original fixture.

Yet truth be told, when I finally caught my breath and reentered the world of normal human interactions, I was appalled and frightened by my capacity to become so completely engrossed in a project that everything else in my life became secondary. I also recognized a definite pattern of moving from one project to the next; and although I fervently expressed a desire to "slow down" to anyone who was still listening, these were in fact empty words, for I was unable to withstand the excitement inherent in a new adventure. I vowed at this point not to take on another large-scale project until my children had reached a stage of greater independence, a promise that I adhered to with steadfast determination.

I have very good memories of this time period, when I avoided hobbies and projects that could spirit me away for extended periods of time. And I believe that the close relationships that I hold with my husband and children can be attributed in part to this change of agenda—which was prompted by the realization that my family did not deserve to be repeatedly relegated to the position of second fiddle, behind a stained glass project or a grand PTA event where Santa was forgotten in the bathroom. For this wake-up call, I am truly grateful.

It would be a disservice, however, to end this chapter with a message that could be misconstrued as: "Hyperfocus is akin to emotional neglect and abandonment." Absolutely not! I encourage my clients to follow what truly interests them so that they can capitalize on the AD/HD capacity to hyperfocus. When parents ask me what areas their AD/HD children should consider when choosing a career, I advise them to support their children's special interests and talents, whatever they may be, because if these children are encouraged to follow paths that hold their interest and excitement, they surely will excel.

However, it is also important to recognize that although the ability to hyperfocus can be a gift and a valuable asset, the capacity to blot out all other aspects of your life can serve as a liability. Hyperfocus is a powerful phenomenon—and I have learned to approach it accordingly.

Chapter 6

Don't Forget to Push the Power Button

In our family, it is my husband who holds things together by maintaining some semblance of a daily routine. It is he who suggests that 10:00 pm is a *tad* too late to make a run to the convenience store with the kids, no matter how much we are craving something sweet. He's the one who proposes that the music be turned down at a "reasonable" hour and that watching late-night cartoons is *probably* not appropriate on a school night.

When the kids were in preschool and he would leave town for short trips, our lifestyle would typically unravel after a few days, and it would not be unusual for the entire family to be in high gear at midnight, lights ablaze in every room, the kids watching their favorite videos, and me, sledgehammer in hand, removing a wall that in my mind was unnecessarily restricting, while listening to old Beatles tunes at top volume.

There was a predictable pattern to these weeks when my husband was away: I would start off the week determined to maintain the daily routines that were already in place. How difficult could that be? By midweek I would be reveling in the fact that schedules were clearly overrated and that "Twist and Shout" might be the best tune of all time. By the end of the week, we would all be exhausted, and I would greet my husband with a hug of sincere gratitude, so very happy that he was finally back and that our lives would return to a state of reassuring predictability and consistent routine.

Although I took full responsibility for the many mishaps that had defined my life up until that point and appreciated (at least in hindsight) the structure that my husband provided, I nevertheless harbored a secret wish that just once he would screw up and forget or overlook something. Finally it happened. My husband and I both bought laptop computers so that we could bring our work home to finish up after the children were in bed. My husband, in his kind but concerned manner, informed me of the numerous ways that I could unintentionally harm my computer, and he reminded me daily of the dos and don'ts of computer maintenance.

And then one morning he woke up and discovered that his computer was dead—completely unresponsive. Of course, he immediately glowered at me with a dark look of suspicion, but I reassured him that I hadn't touched his computer. After all, I had my own that was working just fine, thank you very much! Finally, after interrogating the children and the family pets, my husband came to the conclusion that he must have inadvertently closed the lid to his laptop without powering down the computer.

This was too good to be true! While getting ready for work, I would stick my head in whatever room he was in and say solicitously, "By the way, you need to turn *off* your computer before shutting the lid!" I even called and left a message for him at work with this sage piece of advice, cackling with delight as I hung up the phone. But this was clearly not enough. Then it came to me! I would put a little one liner in the classified section of our small town newspaper, which was composed in a state of amusement that reached near manic proportions: "Bill. Don't forget to push the power button. Cathy."

I should have been a little suspicious when the receptionist in the classified department burst out laughing after the wording of my classified ad was relayed to her over the phone. I tried to explain the whole computer scenario to her, but she didn't seem to buy it. "Hmmm, strange woman," I thought while hanging up the phone. I figured that my husband probably wouldn't even notice the one liner in the multi-page classified section and that it would have to be pointed out to him when it appeared in print.

Over the course of the next day, the classified ad was pretty much forgotten. AD/HDers tend to be engrossed in the moment, and what was centrally important the day before, both good and bad, can be a distant memory after a good night's sleep. Therefore, I was a little taken aback when I received a call from my husband who informed me that my little one liner in the classified section was making the rounds at the clinic where he was employed and that people were coming by, nudging him and saying slyly, "The power button, huh, Bill?"

It was only then that the alternative meaning to my little inside joke registered, and I was appalled. Did my fellow townspeople really think that I would do something so crass? (Apparently, yes.) More important, are there really people out there who read the classified section with such attention to detail? (Apparently so.) Once again, my wonderful, supportive, and long-suffering husband was the victim of my oversights. Poor, poor guy.

Chapter 7

Why the Tooth Fairy Is Always Late

If the Tooth Fairy were scheduled to pick up teeth at a particular time and day, let's say Tuesdays at 7:30 pm, my guess is that the AD/HD parent would rarely forget this important responsibility. Unfortunately for AD/HD adults, this is not the case. My three oldest children grew up with the idea that the Tooth Fairy could not be relied upon to visit on the *exact* night after a tooth was lost. Rather, the tooth might remain under a child's pillow for two or three days before the Tooth Fairy finally made her appearance.

In defense of AD/HD adults who are guilty of this particular transgression, I must say that we truly do not intend to leave little Johnny's tooth under his pillow for three nights straight. We think about the tooth periodically throughout the evening. More accurately, we are repeatedly *jolted* by the sudden recollection that there is a tooth under Johnny's pillow. We are reminded of our duties when Little Johnny goes to bed and gives us that meaningful look as he mentions his tooth and its exact location. We think about it as we brush our own teeth: "Johnny should be fast asleep by now. Let me tiptoe into his room and make the tooth exchange!" And the next thing we know, it is the following morning, and Johnny announces with a disappointed expression on his beautiful little face, "The Tooth Fairy didn't come again last night."

I used to bear this dirty little secret with great shame and could imagine each of my children lying on an analyst's couch in the future wondering, "How could I possibly feel that I was important when my tooth languished under my pillow night after night?" Although the analyst scenario may still be a possibility, I finally came to an understanding as to why I repeatedly forgot something so important in the eyes of my young children, as well as what I could do to remind the Tooth Fairy of her duties in the future.

I have learned from many years of personal and professional experience that the worst possible time for an AD/HDer to remember to follow through on a responsibility is during a time of transition, particularly when moving into an activity that is overlearned and essentially automatic. It appears that once an AD/HDer transitions into this overlearned activity, he or she becomes absorbed in the familiarity of it all, and thoughts that were on his or her mind only moments before are pushed aside and forgotten.

Let's take the responsibilities of the Tooth Fairy as an example. Being a night owl by nature, a common phenomenon for AD/HDers with excess energy, I was assigned the position of Tooth Fairy in our family. Taking this responsibility to heart, I would wait until I was certain that my children were fast asleep before making the swap. I loved the idea that they still believed in magical possibilities and did not want them to wake up to find their mother furtively jabbing something beneath their pillow. It was years before I discovered that none of my children actually believed in the Tooth Fairy and that they went along with the entire charade purely for the monetary benefits.

So although I periodically thought about my Tooth Fairy duties throughout the evening, I typically put off the exchange until I went to bed myself. However, once I moved into my own bedtime routine (brushing my teeth, washing my face, finding nightclothes that did not have the distinctly sour smell of forgotten wash), I essentially would go into autopilot, and my Tooth Fairy duties would be completely and totally forgotten until the following morning.

Although one could argue that fatigue was a factor in my Tooth Fairy failings, I began to notice a distinct pattern of forgetfulness that occurred whenever a task was tacked on to a daily, overlearned routine. If, for example, my husband asked me to return a video on my way to work, once I entered into get-ready-for-work mode, I would go on automatic and most likely leave the video on the counter where it had been strategically placed. If I actually remembered to take the video with me to the car, chances were high that it would remain on the passenger seat, unnoticed and forgotten, as I became absorbed in thoughts associated with driving to work. ("I'm going to miss the green light, *as usual*, because of the idiot in front of me who apparently has all the time in the world.")

As a general rule of thumb, I believe that it is unwise to ask or remind an AD/HDer to do *anything* when he or she is in the midst of a transition. As your AD/HD partner is walking out of the house, do not ask him or her to pick up a gallon of milk on the way home from work. Chances are quite high that the milk will have been forgotten before your partner has turned the ignition key in the car. Likewise, do not remind your AD/HD children as you drive them to school about a change in their after-school schedule. Once they get out of the car, meet up with their friends, and move into the building, your reminder will have been pushed to the far recesses of their minds. If, however, you can sit down together at dinner and plan out what needs to be done the following day, the rate of follow-through will most likely improve. Using *strategically placed* written reminders increases the likelihood of follow-through even more.

Parents often wonder how AD/HD preteens and teens can consistently forget books or assignments in their lockers, but when you look at it from a transitions perspective, it makes all the sense in the world. AD/HD teens may remind themselves repeatedly throughout class that they need to bring home a certain book; yet when they go out into the busy hallway, filled with other students in the process of getting ready to go home, they move into going-home mode, and their thoughts are dominated by this very familiar scene. Perhaps they think about what they will do once they get home—what there is to eat or who they want to call—and the thought of bringing home a specific textbook is completely shoved aside. When they tell their parents, "I forgot!", this does not mean that they don't care or that it wasn't important to them (accusations all too familiar to the AD/HD individual).

Along these same lines, I encourage teachers to remind their students about upcoming homework assignments at the *beginning* of class and allow them a few minutes to jot this information down in their planners. If teachers wait until the end of class to make announcements, I can guarantee you that most AD/HD students will have already moved on in their minds to the between-class mode, and when their parents ask them later about any homework assignments, they will have at best only a vague recollection that *something* is due the next day.

Once I became aware of this particular pattern of forgetfulness, I was able to set up some safeguards to improve my own rate of follow-through. One of the most effective interventions for me has been the use of sticky note reminders that I utilize whenever I need to remember something that is not part of my daily routine. If, for example, I need to pick up something from the store on my way to or from work, I will place a sticky note at eye level on the back door, reminding me of what I need to do. If I am in a particularly foggy state of mind, I will take that sticky note and place it on the steering wheel of my car. Although this may sound pathetic to the uninitiated, I have learned from experience never to assume that I "can't possibly forget" something. These notes provide a certain peace of mind, a safeguard so to speak, against the unexpected daily challenges of AD/HD. (When you live for the moment, every challenge is unexpected, as well as every heartfelt laugh, every beautiful sunset, and every gesture of kindness that unexpectedly warms your heart on a daily basis.)

This same strategy can be used by students to overcome the problem of forgetting key items that need to be brought home from school. Students need to be aware of this potential glitch in their end-of-school routine and have a strategically placed reminder note in their locker that jars them out of their going-home mode long enough to determine what papers and books they will need in order to complete their homework assignments.

Finally, I am pleased to say that I was able to find a way to successfully fulfill my Tooth Fairy duties, and I have not forgotten a single tooth for the past several years. You see, I have enlisted the help of my one daughter who is still of tooth-losing age. When my daughter loses a tooth these days, she leaves a note on the bathroom counter for the Tooth Fairy, which provides a reminder at a critical juncture in my bedtime routine. At this stage in her development, her notes are becoming increasingly sophisticated; and if, heaven forbid, I forget to honor my Tooth Fairy duties one night in the future, she will undoubtedly add on compound interest in her subsequent notes.

This underscores an important message for AD/HD adults. Once you become aware of a problem associated with your AD/HD symptoms, the solutions are only limited by the extent of your imagination. If your first intervention is not successful, fine-tune it until it meets your needs. Don't assume that you *should* be able to function without these accommodations—rather, assume that you *won't*, and act accordingly.

AD/HD truly *is* a disability, and forgetfulness is a prominent symptom of this disorder. Acknowledging the fact that you have a disability does not mean that you are copping out or looking for excuses. Quite to the contrary, accepting a disability perspective of AD/HD is the first step toward purposeful action—finding creative solutions that will allow you to function more effectively and successfully in the future.

Chapter 8

Thar She Blows

In the previous tale of the memory-impaired Tooth Fairy, we looked at what happens to the AD/HDer's mental to-do list when transitioning into an overlearned, nearly automatic activity. For us AD/HDers in such settings, the salience of the familiar routine seems to flood our conscious awareness, and we become completely engrossed in the here and now. What was on our minds only moments before is often shoved aside and temporarily forgotten. (The term *temporarily* is used very loosely here and means that we have not *permanently* forgotten what we were supposed to do—for the most part.)

Transitioning into any highly engaging activity can in fact lead to forgetfulness of the immediate past. Think of times, for example, when you have run into the grocery store on a quick errand ("I'll only be a sec!") and unexpectedly come across a friend or acquaintance in the produce section. Although you may have been on your way home to fix dinner or en route to pick up your partner from work, you become engrossed in conversation and all sense of time and place disappears. Once again, the here and now takes precedence over the immediate past—a bewildering experience for the well-intentioned AD/HDer and a frustrating occurrence for those around us who are impacted by these recurring memory lapses.

What happens, however, when an AD/HDer is transitioning from one engrossing situation to another—when one here-and-now experience collides, so to speak, with another of equal intensity? That is the topic of this chapter.

Imagine the following scenario: You are driving home from work, thinking about what occurred that day—perhaps rehashing a frustrating conversation that you had with your boss or running through a mental checklist of work-related details that you may have overlooked. If you have AD/HD, you not only are thinking about the day's events, you essentially are *reliving* them, a kind of out-of-body experience that is common to AD/HD folks. You are suddenly jolted out of your daily rerun when you realize that you are already pulling into the driveway of your home.

Before you know it, you are opening the front door and—*bam!*—your teenage daughter is telling you about the unfair homework assignment given to the class because her teacher was in a particularly cranky mood. "She's so unfair! Everyone in the class feels the same way. Why should we have to suffer just because she's having a bad day?" Your younger son is competing for your attention in classic AD/HD form: "What's for dinner? Can I have a snack? Sarah had one—I want one too! Can I? Can I, Mom?" No one is quite sure where your oldest daughter is, and you have a vague recollection that she imparted this information to you as you were getting ready for work. Were you supposed to pick her up somewhere? As you are trying to find some memory trace of this important information, while battling intrusive images of your teenage daughter standing alone on a street corner, the phone rings; but the handset, of course, is not in the charger, and you have to plow through piles of papers, books, and dirty dishes that have accumulated on the kitchen counter in an attempt to locate the phone before the caller hangs up.

The caller, it turns out, is your spouse, who tells you that he or she is going to be late and then asks in an aggrieved tone, "Is everything *all right?*" As you wrestle between two competing responses to this asinine question, you become aware of the fact that one of your socks is strangely wet and cold, and you realize belatedly that you tipped over the cat's water dish while dashing to get the phone. Suddenly you hear a voice screaming in the background—no wait, it's *you* that is screaming, and you recognize that you are completely and totally overstimulated. As you continue to yell, a little voice in your head reminds you that you have not seen your children all day and that this is probably *not* the parental response recommended by most child-rearing experts (who no doubt have live-in housekeepers and nannies).

How did you go from a well-meaning parent to a raving lunatic in three minutes flat? Let's review what happened. In this scenario you came home completely absorbed in work-related issues. Without taking a breather, you walked in the door and were bombarded with all the stimulation and intensity of your home life. System overload!

For anyone with AD/HD, I need not tell you how stressful these types of transitions are. You feel as if every nerve ending is on high alert and every noise is magnified. Any demand for your attention, no matter how benign, feels like a full-frontal attack, and you either retreat into the bathroom to regroup (and Lord help any child who knocks on the bathroom door at this point in time) or you blow a fuse, as illustrated in the example above.[18]

Transitions are not the only time that AD/HDers struggle with overstimulation and the angry outbursts that often co-occur. AD/HDers are at risk for emotional outbursts any time there are too many simultaneous demands being placed on them or their environment becomes too intense. These angry outbursts seem to come out of nowhere, although once you become familiar with what triggers your anger, you can recognize telltale signs that you are at risk for a blowup.

Think of the times that you are driving along the highway—music playing, children talking, and all is fine with the world. Isn't it great to be traveling as a family? The next thing you know your turn-off is looming before you and you need to determine, with cars zooming past you on both sides, whether you will be exiting on the right or left side of the four-lane freeway. You make it over to the exit with seconds to spare but now are given the choice of Route 47 East or Route 47 West. How the hell are you supposed to know this? Suddenly, the music is way too loud, and your children's laughter sounds more like the pounding of metal spikes. *"Keep it down for God's sake!"* you hear yourself yelling, and your children wonder what evil alien has suddenly taken over the role of driver. (And no, we didn't map out the trip ahead of time. What kind of question is that?)

There is a thin line between stimulation, which many AD/HDers crave, and overstimulation, which can suddenly send you into a tizzy. As AD/HDers, we *know* when we have become overstimulated—it's very similar to the sensation of sticking your finger into an open light socket. What we need to figure out, however, is what kinds of situations invariably lead to overstimulation and what we can do to circumvent this occurrence.

When my children were younger, the most stressful time of the day for me was arriving home after a long day at work. Although I did not necessarily blow up on a daily basis, I often felt like a bundle of nerves shortly after walking through the front door. A warm and insightful colleague suggested a solution, and it worked like a charm. I determined the halfway point in my ten-mile drive from work to home, a large billboard advertising a restaurant in town. Prior to reaching this particular billboard, I would process my day at work as thoroughly as possible, even pulling over to jot down a reminder of something I needed to do the next day. Once I reached the halfway mark, however, I would force myself to switch gears and start thinking about arriving home, literally *visualizing* what would happen when I walked in the door: who would greet me, what state of disrepair the kitchen would be in, what I would make for dinner, which child would most likely remain in the kitchen to chat about the social events that had taken place at school that day. (Any discussion of *academic* activities would have to be forced out of them through various means of coercion.) By the time I arrived home, I had essentially transitioned over to my home life and could avoid the collision of work and home that often proved overstimulating for me.

Recognizing the early signs of overstimulation is also important. Often times AD/HDers will notice a hypersensitivity to noise and touch when there is more stimulation than they can tolerate. An exaggerated startle response is another warning sign (for example, leaping a foot in the air when someone unexpectedly taps you on the arm or calls you by name). Taking a time-out at this point does wonders for the overstimulated AD/HDer and reduces the likelihood of a subsequent blowup.

Whenever possible, physically removing yourself from an overstimulating environment, even for a few minutes, will allow you the opportunity to calm down and regroup. If that is not possible, deep breathing and tension-reducing exercises are also quite effective. (Drop your shoulders and picture the weight of your day rolling off them. Imagine that your arms are heavy. Let them drop to your sides, down further and further as your shoulders relax. Let your head slump forward onto your chest while you stretch your neck muscles. Breathe in deeply and let more weight roll off your shoulders. Your children, fearing the onset of a seizure, may actually hightail it from the room at this point, removing your source of tension altogether.)

It has been estimated that anger control problems exist for the vast majority of AD/HD adults. Dr. Daniel Amen, in *Healing ADD*, notes that up to 85 percent of people with AD/HD have what he refers to as "rage reactions." I believe that a distinction should be made, however, between "blowing a fuse," a fairly common experience that occurs when an AD/HDer is overstimulated, and "rage reactions," episodes of intense anger that occur with troubling regularity in a minority of AD/HDers.[19] Although both may involve emotional outbursts, the intensity, duration, and quality of emotion are very different. Blowing a fuse occurs when the AD/HDer's threshold for stimulation is surpassed and he or she feels overwhelmed, out of control, and perhaps even a bit frightened by an internal state of chaos. The emotional outbursts that occur at such times are almost a means of counterattack—the AD/HDer's instinctive attempt to reduce stimulation and regain a sense of order and control over his or her environment. Once the environmental stimulation is lowered to a manageable level, the angry mood dissipates as quickly as it developed.

A rage reaction, on the other hand, has an intensity, depth, and red-hot quality and seems to take on a life of its own. Even after you've fully expressed your angry feelings, rage continues to ooze out of you, as if you were some kind of possessed demon. There seems to be a disconnect between rational thought and emotion at such times, and although you are aware at some level that you have made your point (most likely repeatedly) and that your anger is out of proportion to the alleged crime, anger continues to course through your body with frightening intensity. These rage reactions typically are more prolonged than the angry outbursts that occur as a result of overstimulation, and remaining in the situation is most often unhealthy for everyone concerned.

Because of the potential damage that can occur from these rage reactions, finding ways to limit or reduce their frequency and intensity is important. Taking care of yourself, emotionally and physically, will improve your general sense of well-being and consequently decrease the likelihood of a rage reaction. Getting sufficient sleep is critical, since fatigue lowers your resistance to stress and limits your repertoire of potential responses. Exercising regularly is also extremely helpful and allows you to burn off steam and tension that builds up over the day. Eating healthy meals and snacks will avoid nutritional slumps that can leave you in a more vulnerable state.

Finally, for some AD/HDers, these recommendations may not be sufficient. If you find yourself responding with intense anger on a regular basis, there are medications that can be very effective in reducing the intensity and duration of these rage reactions. Individual therapy can also be helpful in terms of uncovering root issues that may have sensitized you to criticism and may be playing a role in your angry outbursts. Gaining a sense of control over your emotional responses is a highly empowering experience, and although this process may take time, the benefits can be far-reaching in terms of your sense of self-worth and the quality of your relationships.

Chapter 9

Learning to Trust the Voice of Caution

One of the best ways that I have learned to help myself as an adult is to trust the little voice in my head that says: "Stop, Cathy! You *will* regret what you are about to say!" When I was younger and even more impulsive, there was a competing influence, the "What the hell—just go for it!" voice; and this voice was far too compelling to ignore. Anticipating the excitement of "just going for it" would often be enough to drown out any thoughts of moderation. After countless early morning self-recrimination sessions, however, I have learned that the "What the hell" voice is invariably *wrong*! Rarely have I woken up the next morning and thought, "I'm sure glad I listened to the 'What the hell' voice last night." Rather, I wake up, cringe with the realization that what I said the night before was not a dream, and think, "Why didn't I listen to the voice of caution? It was *begging* me not to say what was on the tip of my tongue!"

After being swayed by the "What the hell" voice for many years, the voice of caution has become my trusted friend. These are things that experience has taught me: When asked by the hostess of a dinner party what you thought of her new recipe, do not suggest that the flavor could have been enhanced with more salt, even if she says, "I want your honest opinion." Trust me, she doesn't; and your blunt critique will not engender goodwill. Furthermore, sharing that lewd joke that was hysterically funny when your husband told it to you the night before is *not* appropriate at a clinical staff meeting at the local safe house the next morning, no matter how jovial the staff members happen to be at that moment. The jovial mood will end with abruptness. Finally, mentioning the benefits of Prozac as a mood stabilizer is never advisable when talking to your child's teacher, no matter how irate she may be.

I have learned that I do not need to share every thought that goes through my mind, however much I would like to believe that honesty is the best policy.

Listen to your inner voice of caution. With all of the trials and tribulations that you will face as an AD/HD adult, the voice of caution is a trustworthy friend indeed.

Chapter 10

Parenting an AD/HD Child

A long, long time ago (which qualifies in the AD/HD world as any time prior to last month), I attended a local chapter meeting of Children and Adults with Attention-Deficit/Hyperactivity Disorder (CHADD), a national organization that provides education, advocacy, and support for AD/HD individuals and their families. This truly *was* a long time ago, because at that time CHADD's focus was exclusively on issues related to AD/HD in children. This was also before my son or I had been formally diagnosed with AD/HD, and being in an unmedicated state, I was prone to blurting out comments at meetings that I *thought* were relevant, only to lie awake later in the evening, reviewing how truly humiliating the entire experience had been.

I had recently become aware of the statistics concerning the heritability of AD/HD,[20] a whopping 80 percent, which I eagerly shared with the group of assembled parents. "If this is indeed the case," I proceeded without pause, "then a focus of our meetings should be on the inherent difficulties of raising an AD/HD child when struggling as parents with similar symptoms." Rather than the spirited and heartfelt discussion that I anticipated would ensue, my comment was met with complete and total silence, and as I looked around the room in a somewhat confused state, I noticed that everyone had suddenly taken an intense interest in their shoes. Needless to say, no discussion of adult AD/HD *or* parenting took place that evening. I remember lying in bed that night, knowing that I had once again committed a major meeting faux pas but feeling puzzled as to why my comment had been considered so inappropriate by one and all.

That answer was provided for me later that year at a regional conference on learning disabilities, when I had the honor of introducing the keynote speaker, Dr. Robert Brooks, a nationally renowned speaker on issues of learning disabilities and self-esteem. Over the intervening months, I had evaluated many children for learning disabilities and during the process of gathering background information, several parents had confided that they, too, had had similar learning problems when younger. When I would ask if they had shared this information with their children, they invariably would state that they had not and were quick to move on to different topics.

As I waited with Dr. Brooks for the conference to commence, I commented on this reluctance of parents to connect with their children over a shared disability, stating rather primly that students would surely benefit from the knowledge that they were not alone in their struggles. Dr. Brooks, with both insight and compassion, noted how this was an outgrowth of the deep-seated shame that many adults carry with them over their longstanding learning struggles. I was struck by the degree of empathy that Dr. Brooks displayed and recognized with sudden clarity that I, too, had been carrying a heavy burden that came from years of "screwing up." And although I encouraged parents to talk openly with their children about their mutual disabilities, I continued to view my symptoms of inattention and impulsivity as black marks on my character. I was also able to appreciate at a more personal level why no one at that fateful CHADD meeting had leapt to his or her feet and announced, "Hello, my name is _____, and I am an AD/HD adult."

The stigma associated with AD/HD and learning disabilities has diminished quite a bit over the past fifteen years, and parents seem much more willing to speak openly during the evaluation process. The increased acceptance of AD/HD is due in large part to the burgeoning literature on the topic, as well as to the willingness of leading authors in the field of AD/HD to share with their readers that they, too, are coping with symptoms of this disorder.

Included in this body of work are Drs. Hallowell and Ratey, authors of numerous books on adult AD/HD, including *Driven to Distraction* (1994), *Answers to Distraction* (1994), and *Delivered from Distraction* (2005); Drs. Kathleen Nadeau and Patricia Quinn, prolific writers whose titles include *Understanding Girls with Attention Deficit/ Hyperactivity Disorder* (1999), *Understanding Women with AD/HD* (2002), and *When Moms and Kids have ADD* (2005); Dr. Lynn Weiss, whose book titles include *A.D.D. on the Job* (1996), *A.D.D. and Success* (1998), and *Attention Deficit Disorder in Adults* (1997, 2005); Kate Kelly and Peggy Ramundo, authors of one of the earliest popular books on adult AD/HD, *You Mean I'm Not Lazy, Stupid, or Crazy?* (1993, 2006), as well as Sari Solden, MS, LMFT, author of *Women with Attention Deficit Disorder* (1995, 2005), a groundbreaking book that highlights the unique profile of the predominantly inattentive subtype of AD/HD.

Parents of AD/HD children are also more open to the option of being evaluated and treated for their own symptoms of AD/HD, especially as they learn more about how these symptoms impact their daily lives and the lives of their children. The benefits of treating AD/HD symptoms in parents, I believe, are far-reaching. Treatment not only can improve the quality of life for the AD/HD adult but can provide a mental clarity that is extremely helpful when parenting an AD/HD child.

Truth be known, the task of parenting a child who displays the very same features that you are trying to manage within yourself creates a significant parenting challenge. The disorganization that is generated by an AD/HD child can be overwhelming for the AD/HD parent who struggles to find his or her keys each morning. The need to give an AD/HD child repeated reminders may be nearly impossible for a parent who struggles to remember to remind the child the first time around, much less again and again. Having a child dawdle over breakfast can create havoc in the lives of AD/HD adults whose time management skills barely allow them to arrive at work on time when everything goes as planned. This is not to say that the home life of an AD/HD family is by definition chaotic. There are many AD/HD parents who put forth a tremendous effort to maintain a reasonable sense of structure in their homes. This effort, however, is often all-consuming and can contribute to a chronic state of exhaustion for the well-meaning AD/HD parent.[21]

Life can be easier, folks! I speak from experience, having had three children before I was diagnosed and treated for AD/HD.[22] When my son was younger, particularly between the ages of two and five, he could have easily been considered a poster child for the predominantly hyperactive-impulsive form of AD/HD. Given my largely inattentive state of mind, I had a bad record of losing him, particularly in crowded or chaotic environments. (Chaotic was defined at that time as any situation where multitasking was required.)

After my son went missing at a crowded Family Fun Night at the local elementary school (only to be found on a different level of the building, playing happily on the floor with some classroom materials), my husband announced, in a state of anger and frustration, that this was "unacceptable" and "could not happen again." I, with equal indignation, told him that at least our son had not been hit by a car that day, although there were at least two incidences while shopping in which he had tried to dash from the sidewalk into the street. Although the shoe saleslady had to retrieve him as he attempted to scale up the shelves in the back room of the store, at least he was physically uninjured. (I swear I only stopped focusing for a second while I tried on a pair of shoes.) At least he wasn't kidnapped, although there was another point during the day when I couldn't find him because he decided to duck into a rack of clothing as we were walking down the aisle of a large department store. The latter point my husband addressed immediately by stating that if our son were kidnapped, he would be returned within thirty minutes with a note clipped to his shirt which read, "Sorry for the inconvenience and good luck!"

Our ability to laugh about these types of things has gotten us through a lot. We also recognized, however, that parenting an AD/HD child required constant judgment calls and that we needed to establish basic parenting principles to help guide our decisions.[23] An ongoing issue that we were grappling with at that time occurred in the morning when our children were *supposed* to be getting ready for school. Every morning I would tell the children to get dressed and come downstairs for breakfast. Although some days our AD/HD son would be dressed and ready before anyone else, more often than not I would find him half-clothed and deeply absorbed in a Lego building project, having become distracted midway through the dressing process.

When our son was a toddler, I helped him with this morning routine, but when he reached preschool and then kindergarten age, I assumed that he should be able to do these types of things *consistently* on his own. (I, of course, was far from consistent in my morning routine, yet assumed that my five year old should be achieving what I had never to date been able to accomplish.) For a period of time, I tried yelling ("*What are you doing?!*"), shaming ("I have to get myself *and* your baby sister ready, and I thought I could count on you to get dressed on your own."), and even considered sending him to school in his pajamas (an approach advocated by some, but one that I believe is unfair for a child with true time management impairments). Our son would trudge out the door with a look of dejection on his face, and I would begin my work day, as a psychologist no less, feeling like a world-class schmuck.

Clearly, something needed to change. First, I needed to readjust my own schedule so that I could focus my attention on getting the children ready for school, rather than trying unsuccessfully to do more than one thing at a time. (*Multitasking* is a term that was devised to mock AD/HDers: "*Ha, ha, look what we can do that you can't do!*") I also needed to come to terms with the fact that our son was struggling with a disability and that this disability would not magically disappear on his fourth, fifth, or sixth birthday.

Next, my husband and I sat down and hammered out short- and long-term parenting goals. Knowing that the school day is filled with challenges for a child with AD/HD, our short-term goal each morning was to have our son leave for school with a feeling of well-being and a sense of confidence that he could handle whatever came his way. Our long-term goal was to have him reach adulthood with his self-esteem intact and with the necessary skills to function and flourish as an independent young adult.

Lofty goals. So, how does one apply them to everyday parenting decisions? Self-esteem, I believe, is bolstered not only by establishing a home environment that is loving and free of ridicule, but also by encouraging responsibility and mastery in your child. In this manner, he or she can develop both a sense of security as well as self-respect— two basic building blocks of healthy self-esteem. From day one, we have not allowed mean-spirited teasing in our home, and although I've been told by countless grandmother-types that teasing amongst siblings is natural, I'm pleased to say that our home has always been viewed as a safe haven for our children and their friends. To bolster our son's sense of efficacy, however, I needed to step back and determine how to change his environment so that I could give him developmentally appropriate challenges and he could experience success.

Accepting the fact that he was currently unable to consistently remain on task while getting dressed (and knowing that I could not consistently remember to check up on his morning progress), I decided to bring his clothes down to the family room, where I could monitor his progress from the kitchen. "Okay, first take your pajamas off! Hey, that was fast! Good job. Now put on your pants ... Well, look at you! You put on your shirt as well. That's wonderful! Let's get those socks on, and we'll be ready for breakfast!" My son, now extremely pleased with himself, would leave for school with an air of confidence.

"How," the observant reader may ask, "does this dressing procedure lead to your eventual goal of independence? Aren't most four and five year olds able to get dressed without this level of supervision?" Yes, most four and five year olds *are* able to get dressed by themselves, but most children are not struggling with a disability that negatively impacts their ability to remain on task. Placing the same expectations on each of your children, regardless of their level of capabilities, is a recipe for parental frustration and lowered self-esteem in your children.

A second point to remember is that you will not *always* need to micromanage your child's dressing process to this degree. No, you will *not* be doing this when he is in high school. But you will help him to master these tasks *at his own rate of development*, while maintaining his sense of self-worth, so that he is confident when approaching the next set of hurdles along the path of development. It has been estimated that AD/HD children are 20 percent less mature than their same-age peers, and it's helpful to keep this in mind when trying to determine general guidelines for your AD/HD child. Our son is now in a highly competitive college—attending classes, meeting deadlines, succeeding academically, and yes, to set your mind at ease, getting dressed without assistance.

Middle school is a critical juncture for AD/HD students, and it is at this point that the symptoms of AD/HD often become more prominent and intrusive. If you look at the many changes that occur between elementary school and middle school, it's no wonder that many AD/HDers begin to flounder at this time. Suddenly there is a significant increase in responsibility as well as a heavier workload. There is no longer a single teacher to oversee your child's progress, and unfortunately, there is no longer a single desk to contain your child's belongings. Rather, he or she now has to contend with lockers.

The rules of locker usage at the middle school level could probably fill an entire textbook: "Get to school early enough to put your coat and any accessories in your locker. Now take only what is needed for your first class, unless there is not enough time to get back to your locker between your first and second classes, and ditto for the third class. And if you don't bring the right papers to class—there's no going back—just a big zero for you, buddy. At the end of the day, determine which books from your six classes will be required for homework assignments, recognizing that unless you hurry you will miss the bus home, and then you'll be in trouble, although not nearly as much trouble as you will be in if you have forgotten a necessary book, memo, or notepad in your locker." Can you imagine having to deal with this kind of system as adults? We'd all be calling our union reps demanding an immediate change in our contracts!

But such is the reality of middle school. As parents we can sit down with our sixth graders and help them to develop workable systems. Creating a flow chart to put in the front of their binders can be quite helpful, and when your child is rushing from one class to the next, he or she needs only to check this sheet to determine whether or not he or she has retrieved all of the necessary books and papers. Some middle schools have organizational classes for students who are struggling. These classes cover middle school essentials such as filling out assignment books, keeping on top of long-term assignments, taking notes, etc. If your child's school does not have such a program, ask the school guidance counselor for alternative suggestions.

Although your AD/HD child may flounder and need additional assistance when he or she reaches the middle school level, this is also the time to encourage—no, *insist*—that he or she begin to take more responsibility as well. Probably the best possible way to help your child at this point is to teach them the importance of using a planner and writing down all assignments and commitments. From experience, I can tell you that this is much easier said than done.

Initially, many middle school students with AD/HD may need a reminder from their teachers to write down their assignments. But this, I believe, should not extend beyond the first year of middle school. Why? As an AD/HD adult, if you are reminded every time you need to complete a certain task, what happens? Does your need for these reminders lessen? No way! Instead, you heave a sigh of relief and think, "That's one less thing I need to keep track of!" If this occurs to us as adults, why would we expect a different result from our middle school children?

There are many ways, however, that middle schoolers can learn to help themselves. They can set their watch alarms to buzz a few minutes before the end of each class. They can write reminder notes and tape them to the front of their binders. They can also write on the backs of their hands if that's what works for them. If they continue to forget, short-term loss of privileges often does the trick. With our children we implemented a simple system: if the assignment notebook was not filled out, there would be no computer, television, or video game privileges for the rest of the day. It didn't take too long for them to get into the habit of writing down assignments, though I suspect that their friends reminded them from time to time, particularly when a new video game was waiting to be played.

Although certain accommodations are necessary at various stages of an AD/HD child's educational development, other accommodations, I believe, can be more detrimental than helpful in the long run. Accommodations that I routinely recommend at the middle school and high school levels include the option of extended test times (due to the common problem of weak reading retention skills, particularly among older AD/HD students) and the option of taking tests in a less distracting environment. (AD/HD students have great difficulty filtering out distractions, particularly under conditions where higher-level reasoning skills are required.) I also frequently recommend organizational or study skills training for middle school and high school students with AD/HD, as well as teacher-mentors who can monitor AD/HD students' progress on long-term assignments.

Parents have suggested other accommodations, however, that I strongly discourage. Allowing a student to turn in late assignments without penalty is, I believe, counterproductive. Although your AD/HD teenager may tell you that he or she will spend the entire weekend working on a project if granted an extension from Friday to Monday (and at that point they may actually believe this themselves), how often does that really happen? Anyone with AD/HD will tell you that his or her natural AD/HD inclination, if given an extension on a project deadline, will be to put off working on it until right before the new due date comes around. The only thing that this accommodation accomplishes is postponing the inevitable all-nighter! If, however, students are marked down an entire grade for every day that an assignment is late, this will have a greater impact on them and may influence how they approach deadlines in the future.

Throughout the high school years, it is also important for AD/HD students to learn to advocate for themselves. Although it may be tempting to jump in and demand a parent-teacher meeting after your adolescent fails a test, it is more advantageous for students that age to set up appointments with their teachers and to discuss their classroom performance on their own. Dr. Mel Levine discusses the benefits of self-advocacy among high school students in his book, *Ready or Not Here Life Comes* (2005). Levine argues that if parents intervene on behalf of their adolescent children rather than encouraging them to advocate for themselves, "the student is deprived of the opportunity to learn the strategic skills of conflict resolution, stress management, negotiation, and problem solving, all of which are essential in a career."[24]

Guiding your AD/HD child, at his or her rate of development, toward the goal of self-sufficiency is only one of your essential roles as parents. A second and equally important parenting task is to believe in your child's potential and to share this vision with your child. According to Dr. Brooks, national expert on self-esteem in children, one of the most important factors that enables children to overcome adversity is to have adults (parents, teachers, or coaches, for example) who believe in them and who stand by them through thick and thin. As noted by Brooks, "To that end, you can accept your child for who he is, with all his strengths and weaknesses. Whether he's 11, 8 or 5, tell your child often that you love him and show him love in other ways."[25]

One way to show your child that you value them is to spend special one-on-one time with him or her—sharing an activity that your child enjoys. In our busy lives, this may seem like a difficult feat at times, particularly when you have two or more children who desire your uninterrupted focus. But finding a period of time each week to provide undivided attention can reinforce your child's sense of self-worth and help him or her to feel special and valued.

Another way to bolster your child's sense of well-being is to "catch them being good." AD/HD children receive a great deal of negative feedback throughout the day: "Sit down and focus on your work." "Raise your hand before speaking." "Walk—don't run." "Settle down." "Stop bugging your sister!" No one can take this kind of feedback, day after day, and maintain a positive sense of self-worth. Therefore, it's essential that as parents we look for any opportunity to point out positive behaviors when they occur: "Thank you so much for waiting patiently." "That was a nice way to answer your sister!" "Hey, your planner is completely filled out. That's fantastic!" "Thanks for coming home on time. I appreciate not having to worry about you." All children thrive on these types of positive reinforcements, and it's particularly important for children who receive frequent corrections due to their behavior.

Finally, we need to help our children find areas where they excel and encourage the development of these skills. Brooks notes that all children need to have an "island of competency" that allows them to feel good about themselves, and as parents we need to help our children identify their special strengths and to develop them through practice. If it is a skill that they truly enjoy, practice will be something they look forward to, rather than the drudgery that often accompanies talents that parents identify and encourage against their children's will.

In summary, AD/HD is a disability that for many will last a lifetime. *However, AD/HD does not have to be a lifelong handicap.* As a youngster, your AD/HD child will need considerable support from you as a parent to provide a consistent and predictable environment. You will need to recognize your child's weaknesses and work to ensure that he or she experiences success. You may need to go to bat for your child if his or her teacher is unfamiliar with the needs of AD/HD students, and you may need to monitor your child's free time to make certain that his or her environment is not overstimulating. Above all, make your home a safe haven that your child can return to after a long day at school.

It is important, however, for parents to keep in mind the long-term goal of self-sufficiency and not to become stuck in rescue mode. Throughout elementary school the amount of responsibility that you expect from your AD/HD child should slowly increase, and by middle school there should be a clear shift after which your child begins to accept the reality of his or her disability and acknowledges the need for organizational aids. As your AD/HD child progresses through high school, be aware of the fact that the time of eventual independence is approaching and continually assess how prepared your child is for this reality.

Parenting an AD/HD child is not for the fainthearted. But the benefits and rewards of raising a healthy, productive young adult will be well worth your efforts.

Chapter 11

Waiting

In the previous chapter I spoke of the importance of moving your child toward self-sufficiency. My mother has her own unique style.

To: Cathy
From: Mom
Subject: ADD
Monday, 21 June, 7:51

I know you have an ADD problem, but where is your chapter?
Mom

To: Cathy
From: Mom
Subject: Santa
Monday, 21 June, 19:02

You promised—I'm waiting …

To: Cathy
From: Mom
Subject:
Tuesday, 22 June, 7:25
Waiting … goddamn it!

Chapter 12

Smuggles

In the checkout line, Pete embodied the mannerisms of a hyperactive child, squinting at strangers, leaning against the chrome railings, muttering under his breath. Behind him, a couple in their forties exchanged tight, smug smiles. It was smugness, not cruelty, Helen decided, that was the opposite of compassion.

Michelle Huneven, *Jamesland*

Taking the lead from the Harry Potter series, I have developed a new term: Smuggles. Smuggles are individuals who have developed theories of childrearing that are largely unsupportable and are entirely devoid of common decency and compassion. Smuggles are people who smugly believe that your AD/HD child's behavior is solely the result of your poor parenting skills. These individuals also maintain that your own problems with inattention and disorganization could be easily mastered if you just tried a little harder.

I remember having dinner at the home of a Smuggle couple when my AD/HD son was around the age of two. They invited our entire family to dinner, mind you, but then were flabbergasted when our two-year-old spent the abbreviated dinner period in constant motion—moving around the perimeter of their antique-laden dining room, opening and shutting every cupboard door within reach. I do not recall any structural damage—no broken china or splintered doors—which at that time was considered a highly successful outing. It was clear from their facial expressions, however, that an active two-year-old was *not* part of the planned evening entertainment and that when *they* finally had children of their own, they would never allow them to turn into such heathens. (Smuggles are often childless, although there is a subgroup of older

Smuggles who have completely repressed all memories of childrearing and have replaced them with reruns of *Father Knows Best*.)

I spent the majority of the evening trying to entertain our son in an enclosed porch, a room that was out of hearing range and contained no breakables or anything else of interest, while my husband carried on a prolonged (or so it seemed) adult conversation with this couple at the dinner table. I found myself wishing all sorts of horrible outcomes for these newlyweds, including the birth of hyperactive quintuplets with colic that continued unabated for the first three years of life.

That evening was the last time that we were invited to any social function at their home, with or without children. It's funny how having an AD/HD child can bring some long-term relationships to a screeching halt, while cementing other friendships through common experiences, compassion, and a wicked sense of humor about life.

I now view AD/HD children as a true blessing for parents. I use the word *blessing* because I believe that having an AD/HD child gives one the blessing of humility and compassion. Never again will a parent of an AD/HD child pass judgment when they see another youngster who is out of control in the supermarket. Never again will they make smug assumptions that a child's overactive and impulsive behavior is due to the ignorance or lack of involvement of another parent. On the contrary, we parents of AD/HD children need to work harder than the average parent to provide the consistency, structure, and tremendous amount of repetition of rules that AD/HD children need. Even with this effort, AD/HD children will continue to surprise us with impulsive behaviors that we hadn't anticipated or disorganization that we thought we had finally corrected through the use of lists, charts, and repeated reminders.

As parents we play a critical role in the lives of our AD/HD children, for it is our job to protect their fragile senses of self-worth that become deflated by continual reprimands and setbacks at school, home, and in social settings, as well as from a misinformed and condemning public that assumes the AD/HD child is merely under-socialized and is the product of uninvolved or overly lenient parents.

Chapter 13

Taming the Wild Beast

When you read about AD/HD beyond childhood, you will typically come across a phrase that says something to the effect of: "In adolescence, hyperactivity is often diminished and is experienced as subjective feelings of restlessness." Maybe I misinterpreted the meaning behind this phrase, but in my mind the authors seemed to be implying that the high-paced, turbo-charged activity level of the hyperactive youngster becomes *less of a problem* as one matures. Although our high internal tempo may be less obvious to the outside observer and may be seen only in the form of restless legs, tapping fingers, and excessive speech, believe me, these symptoms are merely the tip of the iceberg. Inside of the "hyperactive child grown up" is a churning mass of smoldering energy that is kept under wraps only through considerable effort.

I liken internal restlessness to a smoking volcano. Impulsive speech and fidgetiness are merely outlets to reduce the internal pressure, like a blast of hot steam from a volcano due to erupt. Yes, I probably shifted in my seat a bit more than the average patron at the symphony the other evening, but do you know what I *really* wanted to do? Leap up from my seat and sprint to the nearest exit, screaming: "My God, is this piece really considered music? You could use it in a prisoner of war camp! The mere threat of having to sit through this concerto a second time would be enough to bring the staunchest combatant to his knees!" Apparently, I was alone in this assessment, as the orchestra received a standing ovation from a very enthusiastic audience; although it is possible that some of those standing were fellow AD/HDers who were hoping to get a jump start on leaving the building.

I would argue that hyperactivity does not necessarily diminish with age; rather, through (delayed) maturation and the impact of socialization, AD/HDers eventually gain sufficient self-control to harness the expression of their energy to a greater degree.[26] Surely we continue to show more energy than the average person, often in ways that are not endorsed by Miss Manners. But on the whole, I think we do a pretty good job, given our challenging circumstances.

When I interview other adults with particularly high loadings of hyperactivity, they also describe a sense of physical and mental unease, as if uncomfortable living in their own skins:

> *I get up, run at full speed until I hit my bed sleeping. My mind won't stop thinking of at least twenty things at a time. I can't and don't know how to relax.*

> *I always feel like I've got to go somewhere, where I'm not so sure. It's like a constant restlessness, never quite settled.*

> *I feel that I need to do more than one thing at a time, almost as if I have a motor running at high speed all of the time.*

Many hyperactive adults speak of the challenges of functioning in an adult world with the internal tempo of a rambunctious five year old. With no recess to burn off excess energy, these adults look for opportunities to get out of their seats and away from their desks, and they receive complaints from their energy-challenged colleagues when they shift from one foot to the other in conversation or when they impatiently finish the sentences of those who are speaking a tad too slowly. Even those who enjoy active jobs report negative feedback from their co-workers, who are irritated by the AD/HDers' incessant chatter and overflow of movement.

But when was it determined that plodding steadfastly and quietly through each workday was the accepted norm? I'm inclined to agree with Hallowell and Ratey who state in *Delivered from Distraction*, "Is it really a sign of mental health to be able to balance your checkbook, sit still in your chair, and never speak out of turn? As far as I can see, many people who *don't* have ADD are charter members of the Society of the Congenitally Boring."[27]

Although hyperactivity is a force that requires constant monitoring, when correctly identified and embraced, it can be a remarkable asset to the AD/HD adult. Most successful AD/HD adults capitalize on this internal power source to fuel their varied endeavors, and when correctly channeled, hyperactivity can be a tremendous advantage in the work world. Furthermore, hyperactivity provides us with the necessary energy to cope with the fallout from the *other* symptoms of this disorder, namely, inattention, distractibility, disorganization, and forgetfulness. We *rely* on our hyperactivity when we ransack our home looking for our shoes, when we return to the house for the third time in an attempt to find our car keys, and when we work late into the night on an assignment that should have been started weeks before.

In fact, when excess energy is not available for the hyperactive subgroup to fall back on (for example, when recuperating from surgery or when recovering from an illness), these AD/HDers often experience a sense of being overwhelmed by the many demands that they once found enjoyably challenging, and feel as though their ace in the hole has been taken from them. (This point will be discussed more thoroughly in the next chapter, when we look at the predominantly inattentive subtype of AD/HD, those who struggle with features of inattention, but appear to have less energy than the average person.)

Prior to being diagnosed, however, AD/HD adults can *misinterpret* their chronic symptoms of mental and physical unrest, and the consequences of these misinterpretations are frequently more problematic than the actual symptoms themselves. Let's take a common problem that plagues hyperactive adults, racing thoughts. After a typical day of nonstop activity, AD/HD adults often fall into bed, assuming (or hoping fervently) that they will be asleep within minutes. Although their bodies may be exhausted from physical exertion, their thoughts begin to pick up speed at this point like the Energizer Bunny from Hell.

Before becoming aware of this common AD/HD feature, many adults assume that something must be wrong. Why else would they be unable to fall asleep? So they begin a mental inventory, going from topic to topic in search of an underlying problem that must be causing their internal unease and robbing them of much needed sleep. "Was I too confrontational at the meeting today? Have I missed any deadlines of which I am unaware? Was I attentive enough when my spouse was talking this evening? Should we be going out more often? Am I paying enough attention to my children?"

In this day and age, most adults can find *something* to worry about without too much effort, and over time, the hyperactive AD/HDer may indeed spend an inordinate amount of time worrying over issues that they incorrectly assume are the source of their internal unrest. Yet when anxiety inventories are administered to this hyperactive subgroup, these adults often do not relate to many of the classic features of anxiety and fall far short of the criteria for an anxiety disorder.[28]

Other hyperactive adults assume that their internal restlessness is due to the fact that something is lacking in their lives—as if the excitement is always one town over. Not knowing that they are plagued with symptoms of a disorder, they may begin to question the quality of their jobs or their marriages, and they can be irritable and blaming of others around them. This misperception of internal restlessness can lead to marital tension or relationship problems, frequent job changes, excessive spending, and other impulsive behaviors that are all part of a quest to quell their inner turmoil and to find a sense of contentment. It has been estimated that only 10 to 20 percent of adults with AD/HD have been identified and treated for their attentional problems,[29] and one can only imagine the amount of unnecessary suffering, miscommunication, and misunderstandings that must exist due to undiagnosed AD/HD in adults.

Many AD/HDers turn to substances as a means of calming the raging beast, including nicotine, marijuana, alcohol, stimulants, and cocaine. It has been estimated that approximately 50 percent of *untreated* AD/HD adults struggle with drug or alcohol abuse or dependency.[30] Of interest, AD/HD individuals who are being treated for their attentional problems are no more likely to abuse substances than non-AD/HDers.

Finally, there are some hyperactive adults, often brought in for evaluation by concerned spouses, who are unaware that their energy levels are exceptionally high. Although they may fidget incessantly throughout their interviews, they often deny experiencing symptoms of internal restlessness. With further discussion, it becomes apparent that, having been hyperactive their entire lives, they do not view their supercharged internal tempo as anything but normal. Hallowell and Ratey aptly describe this phenomenon in *Driven to Distraction*: "You can live with something all your life but not be aware of it in its own right; it is simply a part of you."[31]

Things become easier when hyperactivity is correctly identified as a symptom of a disorder. Although we may be reluctant to refer to our high activity levels as "symptoms," once placed in this light, we can focus our efforts on healthy outlets for our excessive energy.

Pharmaceutical interventions can be tremendously helpful in reducing this internal motor for many AD/HD adults. The most common form of psychopharmacologic treatment for AD/HD adults (as well as children) are psychostimulants, and the safety and effectiveness of this form of medication has been demonstrated in over 250 controlled clinical trials.[32] However, even for those who benefit from pharmacologic treatment, oftentimes medication is no longer effective during the evening hours, and therefore additional interventions are necessary.

Second to pharmacotherapy, exercise is perhaps the most effective method of combating overactivity and symptoms of internal restlessness. Whereas non-AD/HDers may choose to exercise to enjoy the increased energy that vigorous exercise provides, hyperactive folks exercise to *burn off* excess energy, as well as to gain a sense of mental clarity and purpose. One client noted that he needs to run several miles each day in order to release some of his pent-up energy; without this outlet, he feels as if he will "go berserk." Setting up a regular exercise program is essential for the physical, mental, and emotional well-being of an AD/HD adult, and finding a no-nonsense exercise buddy, an exercise class, or if possible, a personal trainer will keep you honest and on track.

Deep breathing exercises can also be used to calm the raging beast, and this technique is particularly helpful for hyperactive parents who wish to spend downtime with their children. After becoming quite adept at Lamaze techniques as a mother of four, I began to apply these skills when attempting to relax in the evening. As I sat in front of the television with my children curled up beside me, I would begin to breathe deeply and slowly, letting go of tension with each exhalation. Although the desire to get up to "do one more thing" is initially quite strong, it dissipates fairly quickly when you are determined and consistent in applying these relaxation techniques. Before you know it, you are relaxed and happy, snuggling with your children and wishing the moment would never end. Try it—you may be pleasantly surprised.

Many adults that I have interviewed are unfamiliar with the second form of AD/HD—the Predominantly Inattentive subgroup whose members are often sluggish in their movements, slow to respond, feel easily overwhelmed by stimuli, and need time and space to regroup from daily interactions. This is an often overlooked and misdiagnosed subgroup of AD/HD and is the topic of the next chapter, "And Now a Word from the Inattentive Subtype."

Chapter 14

And Now a Word from the Inattentive Subtype

In the family of mental disorders, the hyperactive form of AD/HD (currently referred to as AD/HD–Combined type) is the bossy older sibling who demands and receives all of the attention, while the Predominantly Inattentive subtype is the younger, quiet child who does not make waves, rarely gets into trouble, but who is also largely overlooked. If you asked the average person on the street to describe a child with Attention Deficit/Hyperactivity Disorder, the vast majority would use terms such as "hyper," "can't sit still," and "hard to control," and everyone could (and would) relate a story about a nephew, sibling, or a little hellion down the street who is "AHDH or whatever you call it." This is the image that is firmly connected to the term AD/HD, and it places the inattentive subtype at a distinct disadvantage in terms of being correctly identified and treated.

The inattentive subtype is, in fact, a relative newcomer to this field of study, and prior to the 1970s, the disorder was defined almost exclusively in terms of hyperactivity. It's not too hard to figure out why hyperactivity was the initial focus of study, and one only needs to stay in an enclosed space with a hyperactive youngster for fifteen minutes or less before the impetus behind these early studies becomes perfectly clear. In fact, I would argue that if hyperactivity wasn't such a thorn in the side of "civilized" society, AD/HD may not have been identified as a disorder at all, and those inflicted would have continued to languish as students in the "not enough potential to warrant serious consideration" category. (Back in the 1960s, through the eyes of a young child, there seemed to be three categories of students: the "smart ones," who were recognized by their hair ribbons, tucked-in shirts, and the ability to raise their hand and *wait* to be called on; the "mentally retarded"

69

contingent, who, according to elementary school folklore, were kept in a room in the basement and were only seen during recess; and the "not enough potential to warrant serious consideration" category, into which the remaining students were lumped, and of which I, and no doubt the rest of the AD/HD contingent, were card-carrying members.)

During the early part of the 1970s, researchers began to recognize that hyperactive youngsters also had a lot more trouble maintaining attention on certain types of tasks than children without hyperactivity, and this prompted an explosion of research that focused on better understanding the various components of this disorder.[33] In 1980 with the publication of the DSM-III,[34] the term *Attention Deficit Disorder* (ADD) was born, replacing the previous diagnostic label of *Hyperkinetic Reaction of Childhood*. This name change was much more significant than what occurs in the advertising industry ("Hey, let's sell the same old stuff under a jazzy new name!"); for it heralded a major reconceptualization of the disorder and acknowledged for the first time the central importance of *inattention* as a defining feature. The DSM-III also identified the presence of a subgroup of ADD that displayed very few signs of hyperactivity, and under the label of "ADD without Hyperactivity," the inattentive subtype was formally established.[35]

Although the diagnostic category of Attention Deficit Disorder without Hyperactivity was first introduced in 1980, it wasn't until the publication of Sari Solden's book, *Women with Attention Deficit Disorder*, in 1995 that the inattentive subtype was brought to the attention of the general public. Solden's description of the inattentive profile was earth-shattering for women who had been struggling with lifelong symptoms of inattention and disorganization, but who understandably could not identify with the AD/HD literature that was based largely on the behavior of hyperactive boys.

In her book, Solden describes how the characteristics of the inattentive subgroup differ markedly from the symptoms associated with the hyperactive type. According to Solden, rather than displaying the classic feature of hyperactivity, members of the predominantly inattentive subtype tend to be *hypoactive*; that is, they are sluggish in tempo and are apt to work, think, and process information more slowly than the average person. Furthermore, whereas the hyperactive individual is prone to impulsive actions and decisions, the predominantly inattentive person often has difficulty moving from idea to action (also known as problems with *activation*). Finally, whereas the ADD individual with hyperactivity is often bored and seeks continuous stimulation, the predominantly inattentive person can become easily overwhelmed when faced with multiple demands for his or her attention. Solden also found in her clinical work that women without hyperactivity tend to shift impulsively from activity to activity and in new life directions, not because of a need for excitement and stimulation, but due to severe disorganization.

For those of you who zoned out during the last paragraph, here's a quick review. (Remember, I promised that I wouldn't make fun of anything that I did not do myself on a regular basis.)

ADD with Hyperactivity	ADD without Hyperactivity
Hyperactive	Hypoactive (sluggish)
Impulsive in behavior	Difficulty moving from thought to action
Easily bored; seeks stimulation	Easily overwhelmed by stimulation

Two very different profiles, wouldn't you say? As one can imagine, inattentive women related strongly to Solden's descriptions, and many felt for the first time that there was a definable pattern to their struggles and an answer to their confusion.

Fast forward fourteen years to the present. What have we learned about the inattentive subtype since Solden's 1995 publication? We now know that an equal number of both women *and* men meet the criteria for AD/HD–Predominantly Inattentive subtype, and that this subgroup accounts for approximately 25 percent of individuals with AD/HD.[36] This means, of course, that the vast majority of both men and women with AD/HD fall into the AD/HD–Combined category. I underscore this obvious corollary because of the fact that articles in the popular press continue to state with alarming frequency that the majority of women with AD/HD display primary features of inattention and few symptoms of hyperactivity.

Solden's observations regarding the low energy level of the inattentive subtype has received considerable support, although when using current diagnostic criteria, *hypoactivity* appears to be present in only a smaller subset of the inattentive subtype.[37] This subset has been named Sluggish Cognitive Tempo (SCT), an unflattering label to say the least, and although the term may accurately describe a defining feature of this subset, unless we are willing to rename erectile dysfunction as Droopy Pee Pees (DPP), it's only fair that we come up a more user-friendly name for the hypoactive subgroup as well. Other characteristics that have been associated with the hypoactive subset include a "daydreamy" quality and social passivity.[38]

Recognizing that the term *inattention* is a multi-faceted construct, current research is also attempting to specify aspects of inattention that are unique to the inattentive and combined subtypes. Although findings on this issue are inconsistent, studies suggest that the inattentive subtype may have more difficulty with selective (or focused) attention, while the combined subtype may have more trouble *sustaining* their attention.[39] Finally, despite a number of experts who suggest that the inattentive subgroup, specifically the hypoactive subset, may represent a separate disorder altogether,[40] researchers are finding more neuropsychological similarities between the two subtypes than differences.[41]

From an observational standpoint, adults in the predominantly inattentive subgroup certainly present very differently than those who fall into the combined subtype, the most obvious difference being the absence of a frenetic activity level. In my practice, when AD/HDers with hyperactivity arrive for their evaluation, they are often out of breath, having attempted to squeeze in a day's worth of tasks before their 9:30 am appointment. They typically speak in a rapid manner, explaining that they have been "hyper" and have had trouble paying attention for as far back as they can remember, but that until recently, they have been able to cope with these symptoms through concerted effort and determination. They go on to describe, however, how their symptoms have become increasingly intrusive and problematic as of late, and they express concern over how this is negatively impacting their work and relationships. (As will be mentioned in the next chapter, the addition of major life stressors can overburden the coping mechanisms of AD/HD adults, who until that point had been coping by the skin of their teeth.)

Despite the intensity of their presenting concerns, there is often a quality of resilience to these adults, a stubborn persistence, and a fighter mentality that have gotten them this far in life. These clients also display an intensity of emotion during the evaluation that is unique to the hyperactive subtype, and there invariably are moments of tears and expressions of regret and disappointment, as well as explosions of raucous laughter and verbalizations of deep-seated relief to have their suspicions of AD/HD confirmed. By the end of the two- to three-hour session, both the client and I are nearly dizzy from the speed at which we covered 143 topics.[42]

In contrast, the inattentive client arrives, often clouded with an air of hesitancy and uncertainty. Whereas it is evident to many of the hyperactive subgroup what their problem behavior has been (having had this spelled out to them by every teacher since the first grade), those from the inattentive subgroup are frequently unaware that they fall into a subtype of AD/HD and seek an evaluation to explore whether or not they have a learning disability or a mood disorder such as depression.

Those who come to their appointments being fairly certain that they have an attention disorder typically have only recently become aware of this possibility and have spent their adult years not understanding why they seem to struggle more than their friends and coworkers with daily tasks and in their pursuit of long-term goals.

As a group, people in the inattentive subtype tend to have more difficulty articulating their thoughts and feelings than those in the combined type, and they report having these types of communication problems in other settings as well. Finally, an overriding feature of this subgroup, particularly in middle age, is one of feeling overwhelmed by the demands of day-to-day life, a characteristic that is much less prevalent in the combined subgroup.

Although I had developed distinct impressions from clinical interviews that I had completed with AD/HD adults, reviewing the literature fueled my interest in exploring the similarities and differences between these two subgroups in a more systematic manner. To this end, I reviewed the psychological reports of 244 adults from my practice who met the criteria for either the predominantly inattentive or the combined subtype of AD/HD,[43] and compiled a list of the most frequently mentioned presenting problems. In addition, when it became apparent upon reading the reports of the predominantly inattentive subtype that the experience of AD/HD changed dramatically once they moved past young adulthood and began to take on the responsibilities of balancing work and family, I further subdivided the AD/HD subtypes into three age groups (ages 18–24, 25–44, and 45–65), and then compared and contrasted their AD/HD experiences between subtypes and across age groups. [44]

The findings were fascinating, both in terms of the similarities and the differences between the two AD/HD subtypes. Given the distinctly different feel of the inattentive and combined subtypes during the evaluation process, I anticipated that there would be significantly dissimilar symptom profiles between these two subgroups. The results, however, confirmed only the axiom that AD/HDers should never assume *anything* based on accumulated memories.

To my surprise, with only a few noteworthy exceptions, there was a remarkable degree of similarity between the two AD/HD subgroups in terms of presenting problems. Adults from both subtypes described similar struggles with sustained attention, disorganization, and forgetfulness. Both subtypes bemoaned their difficulties with reading retention, time management, and attention to detail. And both groups spoke of poor task persistence, describing with equal frequency and intensity the number of unfinished projects that awaited them at home. [45]

The differences in presenting problems between the two AD/HD subtypes, although much fewer in number, were just as compelling in terms of their impact on day-to-day functioning. As would be expected, the presence or absence of hyperactivity is one variable that distinguishes the two subgroups of AD/HD. Whereas only one-fifth of the inattentive subtype reported problems with restlessness, nearly three-quarters of the combined type mentioned internal restlessness as a concern; and the reporting of hyperactivity in the combined subtype did not diminish with age. In fact, one grandfather requested an evaluation because he could not slow down enough to fully enjoy the company of his grandchildren. Impulsivity is a second variable that distinguished the two AD/HD subtypes, and the difference was most pronounced in the youngest age group. [46]

"No duh," says the discerning reader. "Isn't the absence of hyperactivity and impulsivity a defining feature of the inattentive subtype?" Err, yes, so let's move on …

Another intriguing (and less obvious) issue that distinguished the two subtypes relates to the problem of feeling overwhelmed by day-to-day responsibilities. Feeling overwhelmed was a presenting problem that was identified significantly more frequently by the inattentive subgroup than the combined type, and this problem becomes more pronounced for the inattentive subtype during primary childrearing years. In my sample, two-thirds (67 percent) of inattentive men and women between the ages of twenty-five and forty-four reported feeling overwhelmed by their day-to-day responsibilities, compared to a much smaller percentage (22 percent) of adults from the combined subtype.

Feeling overwhelmed is an issue that is frequently addressed in the popular literature, and it is most often discussed in the context of women with AD/HD. Women in our society continue to bear more responsibility for childrearing and housework than men, and the multitasking that is inherent in these responsibilities can exceed the organizational skills of AD/HD adults. Dr. Carol Watkins noted that the lack of structure in the home setting may also contribute to the unique struggles of women with AD/HD. According to Watkins, "Office jobs often have specific schedules and clear job descriptions. The home is much less structured. Tasks may not have a clear beginning or end."[47]

Although I had chosen not to compare men and women in my overall analysis of presenting problems, I was curious as to the degree to which gender played a role in terms of feeling overwhelmed. Are women more likely to feel overwhelmed than men? Further analysis indicated that women from my sample were indeed more likely to report feeling overwhelmed than men (35 percent versus 14 percent), *but both inattentive women and men were more likely to report feeling overwhelmed than their same-gender counterparts in the combined subgroup.*[48] Utilizing the statistical method of odd-ratios, results indicated that the odds of feeling overwhelmed were three to four times higher for women than men in this sample. In comparison, the odds of feeling overwhelmed were *eight times higher* for adults with the inattentive form of AD/HD than adults with the combined type.

This data, although based on a relatively small sample, suggests that it is membership in the predominantly inattentive subgroup that places AD/HD adults at greatest risk for feeling overwhelmed, and that women with the inattentive form of AD/HD are essentially in double jeopardy. This pattern of findings is most pronounced when looking specifically at AD/HD adults between the ages of twenty-five and forty-four.[49] This particular age bracket is unique in terms of its challenges: it is the time that many adults get married, have children, and try to determine a career path that fits their interests and skills. Each of these milestones can be challenging, and attempting to manage them simultaneously is even more daunting. Add the symptoms of inattention, disorganization, and distractibility to the mix, and one can see how "overwhelming" would be a term that is frequently used by AD/HD adults.

But why are adults from the inattentive subgroup more likely to report feeling overwhelmed than those from the combined group, particularly when these two subtypes have so many other AD/HD symptoms in common? Is it possible that without the resource of excess energy, adults with attentional weaknesses are more likely to feel overwhelmed by the impact of inattention and disorganization on their day-to-day lives? Is hyperactivity indeed an ace in the hole or an asset for AD/HD adults? Further exploration into the unique experiences of AD/HD adults with and without hyperactivity is clearly warranted, particularly during the middle- and late-adult years.

A final issue that I would like to address is the impact on the inattentive subgroup of being undiagnosed throughout a significant portion of their adult lives. Because of the vast amount of information on hyperactivity that has been provided by the media, most hyperactive adults who seek treatment these days are aware that they have always been "more hyper" than those around them, and many have a sneaking suspicion that they may in fact have an attention disorder. This is not the case for the inattentive subtype, due to the relative dearth of information on this form of AD/HD. Being unable to meet the demands of adulthood without great effort, being overwhelmed by tasks that seem to be second nature to neighbors, co-workers, and friends, and assuming that any explanation for these shortcomings must involve a damning critique of one's status as an independent and capable adult, is an unbelievable and completely unnecessary burden for inattentive adults to bear.

And so I echo the words of so many authors and researchers in the field of AD/HD: it is of critical importance to educate teachers, parents, pediatricians, and family practice doctors on the symptoms of the predominantly inattentive form of AD/HD so that a timely diagnosis can be made and appropriate treatment can be provided.

Chapter 15

When AD/HD Rears Its Ugly Head

I have many memories of elementary school, although very few of them involve academics. I remember making up adventures for show-and-tell in kindergarten that were more exciting than the reality-bound reports of my classmates, fully convinced that my teacher would believe the unlikely coincidences that were always part of my story lines. I recall having to stand in the corner on a rainy day in second grade when I got caught up in an imaginative story that I was sharing with the girls at my table, which started with a heavy rainfall and ended with their mothers being swept down the street in a torrential current, never to be found again. I can remember being quite surprised (and no doubt tickled) when one little girl burst into tears, and more than shocked and indignant when I was given a stern lecture by my teacher and placed in the corner for the rest of the class period. In general, I recall never being quite sure of what the teachers were talking about throughout elementary school, my mind always flitting off to more interesting topics, such as how little Jimmy was able to chew gum in class and never get caught.

A low point in my acquisition of knowledge came in sixth grade when I was placed next to an autistic boy who spent the entire year spinning a ruler around the point of his pencil. I was as mesmerized as he by the spinning motion, and together we sat in rapt attention. There are definite guidelines to creating a successful spinning motion. If you launch a ruler with too much force, it will take off across the room at a lethal pace; but if launched half-heartedly, the ruler merely wobbles in a most pathetic manner. Class lectures that year took on the following form: "The order of the planets from the sun is … " "Ooh, nice spin!" "And the distance from the Earth to the sun is ..." "Jesus Christ—watch where you're pointing that thing!"

My impulsivity and internal restlessness took a turn for the worse when I hit puberty,[50] and sitting still became next to impossible. My memories of middle school include orchestrating a walkout over the Vietnam War, purposely getting kicked out of class so that I could run home and eat breakfast undetected, and learning how to forge my mother's signature on a long slew of letters that began with "Please excuse my daughter's absence from ..."

As a result, my attendance in high school was monitored personally by the dean of students, an uncompromising man whose stated mission was to teach me that no student was *ever* able succeed unless he or she followed the rules, a philosophy that I spent four years trying to discredit. Although my attendance improved under the dean's watchful eye, I used my excess energy to ferret out the exception to every rule, the weakness of any argument, and the underground passageways to every building on campus.

A particularly acerbic teacher told me during my sophomore year that I did not have a teacher-friend in the school. I don't remember being particularly upset by this comment, more intrigued, perhaps by the unfathomable phenomenon of group unanimity. How can that many people agree on anything? I also knew his comment to be untrue. Perhaps I was disliked by 95 percent of the teachers, but not by all of them, and I'm certain that I informed him of this fact.

My memories of college are somewhat hazy, the result, no doubt, of the severe sleep deprivation that took place over that four-year time span. Although I started each trimester with the best of intentions, I typically procrastinated for the first six weeks of every ten-week term, being lured away from the library by the prospect of having more fun, and then would spend the final month in a state of panic, working feverishly on projects that should have been started weeks before. I was always challenged by the papers and assignments once I started them and berated myself for putting them off for as long as I did. In typical AD/HD form, however, my learning curve was more of a downward slope, and it wasn't until graduate school that I finally got the knack of staying current with the class syllabus.

I certainly can remember my inability to retain what I read (a common and extremely frustrating aspect of AD/HD), and in addition to assuming that I was suffering from an extended existential crisis, I spent many an hour imagining the reactions of my family and friends when it was discovered that I had been stricken all along with a brain tumor. ("My goodness, she did so well considering the fact that she had a tumor the size of a golf ball lodged firmly in the site where all college-related studying takes place.") I am convinced, however, that it was my parents' unwavering belief in my capabilities that provided the impetus to obtain decent grades and fueled my all-night cramming sessions. Their positive regard and high standards must have been internalized because I never considered failing, or even receiving below-average grades, to be an option.

In graduate school, focusing on a subject about which I became increasingly passionate, I was a different student altogether, attending all classes, maintaining a high grade point average, and enjoying a civil dialogue with my professors, who, to my astonishment, held me in positive regard. I've always considered myself extremely fortunate to have found a profession that I so thoroughly enjoy, and I am well aware from my history that I could have become the employee from hell in any number of other occupational settings.

It wasn't until my second son was diagnosed with AD/HD that I began to think more critically about my own attentional skills. I can recall my parents using the term "hyperactive" when discussing me as a child, and I was told that it was my father who refused to consider placing me on medication. Yet I did not revisit this diagnostic possibility for another thirty years, not even when I began to utilize behavior checklists to assess clients for AD/HD on a regular basis. This, I believe, was self-protective behavior at its finest, because when I finally applied these checklists to my own conduct, I was oddly surprised by how overwhelmingly AD/HD I actually was.

I am not alone in my midlife diagnosis of AD/HD; in fact, it has been estimated that the average AD/HD adult is not diagnosed until he or she is thirty-five to forty years of age.[51] And those of us who have been diagnosed are clearly in the minority. As mentioned previously, approximately 80 to 90 percent of adults suffering from AD/HD have not yet been identified or treated.[52]

Much has been written about the various reasons why AD/HD in adulthood is so grossly underdiagnosed and why these symptoms are not recognized earlier in life.[53] What I will be focusing on in this chapter are the forces that finally bring AD/HD adults in to be evaluated, hence the title of this chapter, "When AD/HD Rears Its Ugly Head."

When an adult comes in to be evaluated for AD/HD, we can invariably trace his or her symptoms of inattention and/or overactivity back to childhood. When asked, most AD/HD adults can recall daydreaming throughout elementary school, and many remember having difficulty sitting still in class. Although some describe themselves as "rambunctious" when younger, their behavior typically was not problematic enough to draw attention or raise concern. Many recall being seen as a disappointment to their parents and/or teachers, and their inability to work to their level of potential was viewed as a character flaw rather than a neurocognitive impairment that could be addressed and treated.

Reviewing these clients' histories often reveals patterns of inattention, disorganization, and for many, internal restlessness identifiable at each stage of their development. The child who daydreamed in elementary school evolves into a young adult who daydreams in college or who cannot remain focused in conversation. The youngster who continually misplaced his or her homework matures into an adult who cannot find his or her car keys, shoes, or important insurance forms. And the child who hated to sit still in class is also the adult who can barely sit through the evaluation process, looking as if he or she may bolt from the room at any moment, screaming, "I can't take it any longer! To hell with a diagnosis!"

Yet these self-referred individuals often have admirable strengths that have allowed them to succeed *despite* their attentional weaknesses. I have had the privilege of meeting and working with many, many AD/HD adults who have earned community-wide respect for their occupational achievements, including teachers, physicians, nurses, therapists, judges, lawyers, contractors, entrepreneurs, artists, architects—the list goes on and on. It's important to recognize that although AD/HD creates unique challenges in adulthood, it certainly does not need to preclude adults from pursuing their dreams and reaching their goals.

What then is the catalyst that finally drives AD/HD adults to seek treatment? Many self-referred clients have habitually burned the candle at both ends. A job that would be considered stressful for a non-AD/HDer is even more challenging for an AD/HD adult because of the additional time and effort that is required to compensate for AD/

HD symptoms. AD/HD adults are easily distracted and sidetracked by background noises, and they often have difficulty regrouping and refocusing after being interrupted in their work. Misplacing tools or memos, having to triple-check calculations, and needing to *repeatedly* reread written material are other AD/HD problems that work against productivity and create heightened levels of stress and frustration. Many AD/HD adults will stay late, come in over the weekend, or bring work home to complete in a less distracting environment, which, of course, eats away at family time and provides additional fodder for the late night worry inventory.

Now add one more responsibility, an additional challenge, or one more layer of complexity to the life of an already maxed-out AD/HD adult. These challenges can be positive ones such as the birth of a child, a promotion at work, or for those who are self-employed, a significant increase in business. More stressful challenges include returning to school, relationship concerns, or the arrival of one's AARP membership application. Suddenly the demands of life exceed the coping mechanisms that have worked for these adults to date, and AD/HD symptoms seem to attack with a vengeance. Competent professionals report being unable to walk from one part of the house or office to the other without forgetting what they were planning to do, and when they come in for an evaluation, they typically feel as though they are hanging on by a thin thread. Hitting the proverbial wall is a common precipitant that leads AD/HD adults to seek treatment.

Another challenge that significantly impacts the coping mechanisms of AD/HD women and deserves special mention is the onset of menopause. There is an association between levels of estrogen and the severity of AD/HD symptoms. The higher the level of estrogen in a woman's body, such as during pregnancy and while breastfeeding, the fewer the AD/HD symptoms. But now for the bad news: lower levels of estrogen lead to a worsening of AD/HD symptoms. Here's a direct quote from the 2003 National Women's Health Report on AD/HD across the lifespan: "The lower the levels of estrogen—just before your period, and just before, during, and after menopause—the worse the symptoms."

Now, wait a minute! I'm not comfortable with the "and after" part of that statement. Are post-menopausal AD/HD women doomed to walk around with Post-it notes stuck to the fronts of their shirts for the rest of their lives? Why is this not considered a health concern of highest priority? Where is the presidential task force that is addressing this issue?

AD/HD women who seek treatment in their mid to late forties present with a remarkably similar set of circumstances. Their story goes something like this: "I have always had a lot of difficulty with organization and time management, and for as far back as I can remember, it has been very hard for me to pay attention. Yet I was able to raise three children, work full-time, and volunteer for various organizations. Over the past six months, however, I feel like I am going nuts. I can't remember things from one minute to the next. I have missed important meetings—I even forgot about my daughter's piano recital, and I had it written down on my calendar! I ran out of gas on my way home from work last week because I kept forgetting to fill up the tank, and my house is in complete shambles." At this point I ask whether or not she has been experiencing any pre-menopausal symptoms. Bingo!

These symptoms don't just pop up around the time of menopause. There is also a dreadful phenomenon called perimenopause, which can start anywhere from two to eight years before the real thing. Maybe everyone else knows about perimenopause, but I was PID (Perimenopause in Denial) for many years and only heard about it while attending a lecture series on AD/HD symptoms across the lifespan. Suddenly I am being told about perimenopause, with all its horrible features like memory loss, lack of mental clarity, word-finding problems, and … umm, you know, what's that thing called? It's kind of frightening to have AD/HD and find out that it's only going to get worse. I guess we can call this "hitting the hormonal wall."

The one good thing about perimenopause and menopause is that non-AD/HD women can get a taste of what we AD/HDers have lived with our entire lives. It's only too bad that men don't go through it as well. The frightening thing about these hormonal changes is that they wreak havoc on the lives of AD/HD women. It's like entering a super-AD/HD state, and it's not pretty.

If you are an AD/HD woman in your forties and are relating to this tale of woe, talk to your obstetrician or internist to determine if they are familiar with treatment issues regarding AD/HD and hormonal imbalances. Even if you are currently being treated for AD/HD, check to see whether or not your medication level needs to be adjusted.

For young adults, the most common reason to seek treatment is a decline in grades toward the end of high school and/or below average to failing grades in college. This particular group of AD/HD individuals has also hit the wall—in an academic setting—and their AD/HD symptoms suddenly are threatening to preclude further advancement.

Perhaps the most intrusive and disturbing manifestation of AD/HD for high school upperclassmen and college students is the almost universal problem of weak reading retention skills. For those readers with attentional deficits, I need not explain the incredible frustration of trying to read material that is less than riveting. You sit down with every intention of reading a difficult chapter, an instruction manual, or even a short newspaper article, and after five minutes you realize that you have *absolutely no idea* what you just read. So you start once again, determined to focus on the reading material, only to discover that although your eyes have been diligently following each line of text, your mind has wandered off again like an errant school boy. Many adults need complete silence in order to read and retain written information that is particularly dense or complex, and even with this luxury, they often resort to reading aloud, underlining practically every word on the page (which kind of defeats the purpose), or giving up in frustration. (Unlike adults with a bona fide reading disability, adults with AD/HD often have no difficulty focusing in on novels or other enjoyable reading material, and they can become so immersed in their reading that they completely tune out others in their environment.)

Although reading retention is a common and vexing problem for most AD/HD adults, it can be a debilitating handicap for college students who do not have the luxury of reading lengthy assignments three or four times before the information finally sinks in. Reading retention problems can also negatively impact test taking, particularly when students are given test questions with "a lot of words." Minor distractions in testing environments (nearby throat clearing, pencil tapping, heavy breathing, or creaking chairs, to name just a few) will further exacerbate reading retention difficulties and invite intrusive homicidal fantasies. Add mounting test anxiety and the effects of sleep deprivation to the mix, and it's not surprising that so many young adults with AD/HD struggle to maintain decent grades at the college level.[54]

In addition to reading retention difficulties, many students who enter college are not prepared for the responsibilities that will fall squarely on their shoulders. To begin with, AD/HD students often fail to develop effective study habits while in high school, and they tend to procrastinate and then rely on last-minute cramming for tests and long-term assignments. Although this approach allows many talented AD/HD students to breeze through high school, it often proves to be ineffective at the college level, where the amount and complexity of the material far exceeds what AD/HD students are able to memorize over a short period of time.

In addition, the number of potential distractions that exist in a college environment can be mind-boggling for even the most organized and focused student, and can be overwhelming for the hapless AD/HDer. Without parents present to set limits, many AD/HD students are drawn to the stimulation that these distractions provide, putting off until later what may be due the next day. Distractions, coupled with a short attention span, also negatively impact a student's effectiveness when they finally *do* settle down to study. One frustrated AD/HD student lamented, "I have a terrible time focusing for more than thirty seconds. When it comes time to do homework, what my classmates accomplish in one hour of studying usually takes me eight hours or more."

Although the challenges at the college level are significant, they clearly are not insurmountable for students with attentional weaknesses. At this stage of maturation, students have the capacity for meta-cognition, that is, the ability to think about how they problem solve. Being aware of one's attentional weaknesses and their impact on day-to-day functioning is critical at this level.

To promote increased self-awareness in this regard, I have developed an inventory that I provide to college students, and I encourage them to assess their behavior as objectively as possible:

- Do you focus better at certain times of the day than others?
- Does your focus improve when sitting toward the front of the class?
- Are you better able to focus after exercising?
- Can you study in your dorm room or must you find a place with fewer distractions?
- Does your understanding of written material improve when you read aloud?

- Do you find yourself overwhelmed by multiple tasks—not knowing where to begin?
- Do you lose track of time or misjudge how much time is required for certain activities?
- Do you procrastinate excessively on assignments?

When a student can begin to pinpoint the types of settings that are most conducive to learning and can recognize their particular areas of vulnerability, they tend to be less overwhelmed by the college experience and become more effective in managing their responsibilities.

In addition, most colleges and universities have excellent academic support services or resource centers available to AD/HD students *who have been diagnosed and have an evaluation that verifies the extent of their disability.* Evaluations are only considered valid for three years—no college will accept an evaluation of your child that was completed when they were in elementary or middle school!

A thorough evaluation must include intellectual and achievement testing to rule out a learning disability, mood inventories to determine whether or not depression or anxiety are contributing to a student's attentional weaknesses, as well as AD/HD inventories to assess for the presence and severity of AD/HD symptoms. The evaluation should also include supporting information from a parent or guardian, and if available, information from previous report cards and/or prior psychoeducational testing. Finally, in addition to confirming a diagnosis of AD/HD (as well as possible co-existing disorders), a helpful evaluation should include classroom accommodations as well as recommendations to assist the student in developing more effective study skills.

Recommendations that I routinely offer to assist students at the college level are listed below. It should be noted that classroom accommodations will need to be requested through special service programs that exist at every college and university, preferably before the onset of the school year.

Classroom Accommodations

1. Reading retention difficulties will increase the amount of time that a student requires in order to comprehend written test

material. For that reason, extended test time should be an accommodation available to students with AD/HD.

2. Given the problem of distractibility that is inherent in AD/HD, students should be given the option of being tested in a separate room where distractions are minimal.

3. AD/HD students should also be given the option of taping class lectures.

4. Individuals with AD/HD very often have difficulty dividing their attention, and this is most noticeable when attempting to listen to class lectures while simultaneously taking notes. Teachers can assist students with note-taking problems by providing "guided lecture notes." These notes are essentially a skeletal outline of the teacher's lecture, with key points marked. Spaces should be provided between each point so that the student can write additional notes. Individuals with attentional weaknesses also have difficulty identifying major themes, and they can become lost in poorly organized and conceptualized details. Guided lecture notes also assist students by identifying the central themes of newly learned material. In addition, these outlines allow a student to get back on track if he or she momentarily loses focus.

5. AD/HD students benefit from regular contact with an academic advisor who can assist them in managing long-term assignments and who can help them to develop an organizational system to effectively juggle the demands of multiple classes.

The remaining recommendations have been found to be helpful at the college level and are directed to AD/HD students themselves:

Recommendations to Improve Organization/Structure

1. Using a daily planner and writing down all assignments is essential for anyone with attentional deficits. Check your planner several times throughout the day. The busier you are, the more likely it is that you will forget appointments and commitments.

2. List making should also become part of an AD/HDer's daily routine. List making is the first step in the process of organizing your life, and it serves several purposes. First, a list can clarify and organize your thinking, particularly if you are suddenly feeling overwhelmed by all of your responsibilities. Lists can help to prioritize projects that need to be completed. ("Hand in term paper" should come *before* "Pick up keg for party.") To make a list useful, however, it must be handy, and it should be referred to frequently.

A note of encouragement: The inability to maintain an organizational system is extremely common for those with AD/HD. Rather than berating yourself over this lapse in attention, you must learn to recognize the telltale signs that you are about to enter into a state of chaos. Don't go there! Catch yourself before you become overwhelmed, make a list of everything that you need to do, and then reinstitute your organizational plan.

Classroom Strategies

1. Sit toward the front of the class. This will reduce potential distractions.
2. When recording a class lecture, carefully label each recording (for example, "Intro to Psychology, 09/15"). Set the timer to zero, and if you are unsure of a concept during the lecture, jot down the time displayed on the recorder in your notes for easy review and clarification later.
3. Attend classes regularly. Although some students can get away with missing class from time to time, AD/HDers cannot. Given the reading retention problems that plague the AD/HD population, receiving information from auditory channels will be most helpful.

Study Techniques

1. Review tapes and/or notes as soon after the lecture as possible. At this point the information is still fresh in your mind, and this will help to consolidate the material and transfer it to

long-term memory. Copy notes over, if necessary. Highlight major points.

2. When reading a textbook, you will find it very helpful to review the chapter overview and the paragraph headings before reading the chapter itself. This is a somewhat time-consuming and difficult process for individuals who are prone to impulsivity and impatience. However, this process will help to create a general framework into which specific facts can be placed. Individuals with attentional weaknesses are much more likely to remember information when it is placed within a larger and more meaningful context.

3. When reading, stop after each section and quiz yourself about what you have just read. Pretend that you are explaining the information to a friend, and as you attempt to do this, you will discover whether or not you truly understand the material. If you have not retained a sufficient amount of information, then you will need to return to the material and attempt to learn it in a different fashion. Perhaps you will need to read the material aloud. Other successful techniques are to diagram the material or to write notes. Highlighting important points can also be very helpful.

4. When studying, AD/HD students benefit from the use of ear protectors or sound cancellation devices to muffle external noises. This intervention markedly improves one's focus and is highly recommended.

5. Take small steps. Frequently, a large project can appear overwhelming, and the tendency of many AD/HDers is to ignore or push away what feels overwhelming to them. Therefore, large projects of any kind should be broken down into manageable components. Rather than thinking about the dreaded project as a whole, tackle one piece of the project at a time. The sense of accomplishment that you enjoy after completing one step will spur you on to tackle another section. Suddenly, the dreaded project no longer seems as overwhelming, and you can enjoy the wonderful sensation that comes from overriding internal objections and accomplishing a difficult feat.

6. Take short breaks while studying, but determine what breaks work best for you. Perhaps a brisk walk outside or a quick trip to the snack bar is what is needed to revive you. Or maybe a short visit to a friend down the hall. You may just want to veg out to music or play a few games on the computer. Frequent breaks will revitalize you. However, if you notice that the quick visit to your friend's dorm room invariably ends up in an evening of debauchery or that computer gaming has a way of transporting you for hours at a time, find other outlets that can be more easily managed! Setting a timer may be a helpful reminder to return to the task of studying. Having *diligent* study partners can be quite effective as well. Then reward yourself when your study session is finally over!

Chapter 16

And What Did You Do Today, Dear?

I considered naming this chapter "In Honor of the Unsung Heroes" because in the AD/HD world, mothers and fathers who are full-time homemakers are exactly that. But AD/HD adults are more likely to identify with the current title, since this is a question that many of us have grappled with at the end of a long day at home. And although we may have worked feverishly on 101 projects throughout the daylight hours, as we stare at the chaos spilling out of each and every room of our homes, we are suddenly bewildered in terms of how indeed our time was spent. Why are time management and task completion such a struggle for AD/HDers, particularly in the home setting?

Sari Solden's description of the expected duties of a homemaker offers insight into the unique struggles of AD/HDers within the home. In her book, *Women with Attention Deficit Disorder*, Solden writes a fictional ad that lists the expectations placed on homemakers:

> Woman wanted to coordinate multiple schedules in an unstructured, distracting atmosphere. Must be able to process great numbers of details quickly and maintain a neat, well-organized environment. Must keep track of all important occasions, including social obligations, birthday cards, and thank you notes, as well as be responsible for all subtleties and niceties of life. Must be able to choose quickly and easily from a great number of options. Applicants will be responsible for all recordkeeping and for maintenance of all systems in the organization, as well as the upkeep on all equipment.
>
> For those interested, please call 911-N-O-T-A-D-H-D.[55]

My guess is that if such a job existed outside of the home, no AD/HDer in his or her right mind would apply for it, for it requires skills that are precisely most difficult for those with attentional impairments: organization, sustained focus, multitasking, and the ability to tune out distractions.

Let's take multitasking as an example. Multitasking is the current catchphrase to describe the process of dividing one's attention and working on more than one project at a time. By definition then, multitasking necessitates the ability to actually *remember* what tasks you are in the midst of completing, a requirement that excludes most AD/HDers from the get-go. AD/HD adults are more likely to become wholly absorbed in one task, until we are distracted by the reminder of another responsibility that really should have been taken care of the day before, and this new task will dominate our attention until the phone rings and we become immersed in conversation, no longer conscious of the multiple tasks that are in partial stages of completion (including the cookies in the oven and the sink that is rapidly filling up with water). In this manner many AD/HD adults spend their days moving from one unfinished task to the next, always in motion, but with little sense of accomplishment by day's end. As one frustrated homemaker stated, "Sometimes I feel just like an AD/HD commercial: one frame or phase after the other, but NO SONG."

Being at home also has a strange way of warping time. Without a work schedule, time seems to melt away. You have only just seen your children off to school when they are suddenly tromping back through the door again. This is most likely due to the AD/HDer's ability to become lost in thought or absorbed in projects. For a while, I set an hourly alarm on my watch, hoping that this little reminder would help me to be cognizant of passing time and allow me to remain present for the fifty-nine minutes between alerts. This intervention didn't work out as planned, but it did allow me the hourly thrill of recognizing how easily AD/HDers can be transposed to another dimension.

Although it would be just dandy as a homemaker to be able to establish a schedule to accommodate all of the tasks that need to be completed in a given day, there are always unexpected interruptions in the life of a stay-at-home parent. Though you may *plan* to organize the bills on a given morning, you don't anticipate that your child's kindergarten teacher will call to announce that little Katie has vomited all over the classroom sand table and ask if you would *please* come pick her up as soon as possible? You also don't foresee that your sewer system will suddenly back up, with foul-smelling toilet water rising ominously close to the rim. And while fielding calls from telemarketers intermixed with reminders from helpful PTA members about upcoming events, you have to wonder if there are any *paid* positions that have these kinds of job requirements.

Suddenly it is 3:45 pm, and your older children arrive home from school with special needs ("I need to get some papier-mâché to make a model of the solar system that is due tomorrow.") and expectations ("My teacher wants you to call her—I'm not exactly sure why."); and before you know it, it's dinnertime, minus the prepared dinner, and your spouse is asking you, like clockwork, what you did that day.

But full-time homemakers are not alone in these struggles! After reviewing hundreds of stories from AD/HD adults, I want to go on record as stating that although many AD/HDers report being more organized and productive while at work, not a single adult stated, "Well, my workday is a complete disaster, but let me tell you about the wonderful organizational system that I maintain at home." AD/HDers who function well within the structure of their workplace describe the chaos that ensues on their days off. AD/HD adults who enjoy a sense of accomplishment during office hours speak in hushed tones about the many unfinished projects that await them at home, how they feel pulled in multiple directions, and how they can't seem to accomplish anything outside of work. As one client aptly put it, "At work I am able to shut all the doors and focus on one thing. At home, too many doors are open."

In the next chapter, I will offer recommendations that may assist you in providing greater organization and structure to your home life. All I really want to say in this chapter is this: Those of you who stay at home have a really tough job, and you should be recognized for the daunting tasks that you take on day after day. Furthermore, you *definitely* should not be hard on yourself. Ask any career-oriented AD/HDer to switch places with you, and he or she will be begging for mercy by week's end. Most important, make sure to take some time for yourself each day to rejuvenate—guilt-free. You deserve it.

Chapter 17

Once You Accept Your Limitations, the Solutions are Limitless

Perhaps as a reader you are part of the large group of adults who have lived with symptoms of inattention, disorganization, and for many, restlessness throughout their lifetimes, but are only just beginning to question whether or not these "idiosyncrasies" are actually part of a larger disorder of attention. You are embarking on an exciting journey of self-discovery. But first you need to confirm your diagnosis. Talk to your parents or siblings and gather more information about your behavior and attention span as a child, as well as about other family members who may have had similar issues. Do you have access to your childhood report cards? These can provide a wealth of information, particularly the sections where teacher comments are located. "Exercises self-control," "listens courteously," "works independently and is not easily distracted," "completes work on time"—these are often areas where AD/HDers receive checkmarks indicating a need for improvement. Next, find a psychologist, psychiatrist, family practitioner, or internist who is well-versed in AD/HD and who can determine whether or not you indeed meet the criteria for this disorder. Talk to your physician about treatment options.

Perhaps you are part of the minority of AD/HD adults who have recently been diagnosed. Receiving the diagnosis alone is often a huge step for adults who have been struggling with these symptoms for as far back as they can remember. So you are *not* immature, self-focused, self-destructive, and all the other negative labels that have been ascribed to you over the years, whether by yourself or by others. Re-labeling your behaviors as symptoms of a disorder is an emotional undertaking. Often AD/HD adults have internalized a lot of negative messages, and they replay them every time one of their symptoms is displayed. "Interrupting again, huh? Are you ever going to grow up?" "Feel like you can't keep up with the conversation? Maybe you should have paid more attention in school." The first step in recovery is to tell these internal bullies to shut up. Yep, and that feels really good. "Shut up! That was impulsivity, not immaturity, and rather than beating myself up over this, I am going to figure out how to best handle these symptoms."

Usually there are a lot of old tapes that need to be identified and then altered. Listen carefully. These tapes have often been playing in the background for so long that you have automatically come to accept their damning judgments. Confront these messages when you become aware of them, and make a decision that you are no longer going to be at the mercy of their negativity.

The next step is to take inventory of how AD/HD symptoms are impacting your life. Are you chronically late for appointments and get-togethers? Do you have trouble relaxing after a hard day at work (or at home)? Do you feel overwhelmed when faced with a large project, and do you consequently procrastinate on getting started? Are you always looking for items that you have misplaced? Be honest with yourself. The purpose here is not to place blame but to look at areas of your life where you need to intervene and find solutions to aggravating behavior patterns.

Now pick a behavior that you would like to focus on first. What solutions have you tried in the past to deal with this? What worked and what did not? For an intervention that did not work, think about why not. Let's take forgetfulness as an example. Perhaps you have tried making lists but didn't find this to be helpful. Why not? Did you misplace the lists? Did you feel discouraged by all the items on your lists? Did you forget to use your list after the first day of this intervention? Don't worry. I'm not going to accuse you of making excuses. These are all legitimate reasons why many people stop making lists. Once you determine *why* list-making was not successful for you, then you can fine-tune your approach so that it *can* work.

In this chapter I would like to review some of the most common roadblocks that are created by AD/HD symptoms and what interventions have been helpful to other AD/HD adults. Some recommendations will hit the mark for you, while others may not. We are all very different, despite our similar symptoms of inattention. Even the recommendations that sound promising to you will need to be tailored to meet your specific lifestyle and circumstances.

Organization

- Without question, a personal organizer as well as a family calendar are essential for all AD/HDers to maintain. Family wall calendars can keep track of all school events, dentist and doctor appointments, vacation dates, visits from relatives, get-togethers with friends, etc. Hang it in a central location like the kitchen so that you can write down events when you schedule them by phone or when you review your children's notes from school. Encourage your children to write down events as well so that there are no last-minute surprise conflicts in the family schedule. Check your calendar before going to bed at night to make certain that you are aware of upcoming events.

- Most occupations will also necessitate a planner to keep track of all the details of work, and this is where personal organizers come into play. Finding a planner or organizer that works for you is essential, and the number of planners that I have purchased and then shelved is an ongoing source of amusement for my family. If a planner is too big and awkward, you will not be likely to bring it with you. If it's too small, you will never be able to cram everything you need to remember on the tiny pages, and even if you could, you'd never be able to decipher what you wrote.

  Then, of course, there are the personal digital assistants (PDAs) that offer a large number of organizational benefits, if you have the patience required to punch in the letters and numbers. Many AD/HD adults do not—and it's an expensive lesson to learn. However, as these handheld computers become more and more sophisticated, they will likely become more AD/HD friendly as well. They also fit in your pocket, a big plus in terms of having your agenda readily available.

- Personal planners are also helpful for those adults who are full-time homemakers, because they can assist you with time management as well. Many AD/HD adults take on too much—and then feel as though they spend their time putting out fires. A well-used planner can assist AD/HDers in not overbooking their days. If you are planning on paying the bills on Tuesday, schedule that activity in your planner, marking off the time as you would a scheduled meeting. If you need to pick up supplies for a school project, put that down as an after-school activity for you and your child. In addition to all the other events that fill up your days, also mark off time for yourself, whether it is to exercise or to chill out and regroup. Once you get into the habit of using your planner in this manner, when you get a call asking if you have the time to help out, you can check your schedule and make an informed decision about whether you have the time or not. If your schedule is full, say no!

- To-do lists are also essential for the busy AD/HDer, and the more you utilize and rely on them, the less likely you are to misplace or forget about them altogether. Knowing that I would be unable to keep track of both a to-do list and an agenda, I combine the two and choose planners that have space set aside for lists. Highlight anything that has not been completed and add it to your next day's to-do list. If you are at your computer on and off throughout the day, another highly effective system is the use of an ongoing to-do list that you can keep in an open folder on your computer. Every time you think of something that you must do, double click your "To-Do List" icon and write it down. You can always print up your to-do list to take with you when you leave the house.

Short-Term Memory Problems

First and foremost, don't assume that there is *anything* you cannot possibly forget! If distracted, what was centrally important to you may be pushed off the radar screen. Interventions that have made my life a whole lot easier include:

- Ask receptionists to call you to remind you of upcoming appointments. Usually they are more than happy to do this and avoid having a no-show.
- Ask friends who call to remind you why they called before they hang up.

- Ask others to write down requests that they have of you, both at work and at home.
- If you need to leave a project midway, leave yourself a note stating where you left off and what you need to do next.
- If you have an item that you need to bring with you, put it next to your car keys or your shoes so that you cannot possibly forget it.

Task Management

- Oftentimes, a large project that needs to be completed can appear overwhelming. Thus, it is strongly recommended that any large project be broken down into smaller components. Create a checklist of steps that need to be completed. This allows you to judge your progress and provides a sense of gratification as you check off item after item.

- Along the same lines, if there is a task that you find yourself avoiding, approach it in short time intervals. Commit fifteen minutes to the task, take a five-minute break to reward yourself, and then commit another fifteen minutes. Pretty soon you will find that the onerous task has been completed.

- Having a large number of smaller tasks to complete can also feel overwhelming, and under these circumstances, AD/HDers often find themselves spinning their wheels, unable to get anything done at all. When you become overwhelmed by the number of tasks that must be addressed, sit down and make out a list of everything that must be done. Include everything that's preying on you; they all take up space in your beleaguered brain. This process allows you to clear your head so to speak, and everything that you need to complete is summarized before you in written form. Now prioritize what needs to be done immediately, what must be done before the end of the business day, what should be completed before tomorrow, next week, etc. Suddenly, rather than feeling overwhelmed, you have an action plan. As you complete each task, the feeling of being weighed down will lighten, and you will feel more empowered.

Sleep/Arousal Problems

- Melatonin, a natural sleep agent, is very helpful in promoting sleepiness, and there is no grogginess the next morning. Take it thirty to forty-five minutes before you want to fall asleep.
- Hot baths or showers are wonderful sleep enhancers.
- Stay off the computer or Internet late at night; those activities are too stimulating and will deprive you of needed sleep.
- Try to avoid taking cat naps because this further interferes with a normal sleep pattern.

Emotional Lability

- AD/HDers can be a moody bunch, and there are times where there may be no true precipitant to an angry mood. Rather than trying to find the causes for one's anger at the world, recognize that the foul mood will pass and limit interactions with others until it does. Learning to laugh at oneself during these foul moods can be helpful as well.
- Although increasing one's organizational skills should be a goal for an individual with attentional weaknesses, it is equally important to allow some time each day to relax and pursue an enjoyable interest. Schedule downtime for yourself; don't wait until you feel overwhelmed.
- Finally, maintain a sense of humor about the situations that you find yourself in as a result of your attentional weaknesses. Although medication and organizational techniques will help to reduce your attentional difficulties, they will not disappear, and you need to accept this unique facet of your personality with a sense of tolerance and humor.

Chapter 18

And In the End

At this point in my career, I am seen as being "in touch with my inner child," and it has been said that I use this "gift" to reach out to child clients and communicate with them at their level. Truth be known, the child within me has always been a dominant part of my personality (formerly known as immaturity)—voicing new perspectives, allowing mind travel, seeing the absurd in almost anything. This, perhaps, is the coolest aspect of having AD/HD. Kids are way cool.

For adult clients who have internalized the negative messages that they received as children (that they are irresponsible, immature, self-centered, and inappropriate) and who are struggling with longstanding issues of shame and guilt, I encourage them to bring in pictures of themselves as children—and to look into the eyes of the child staring back at them and recognize that this child was not "bad" or uncaring of the feelings of others. Rather, they were trying to fit into a world that somehow marched to a different beat than they did.

And I encourage AD/HD adults to get back in touch with this child, to embrace this child. Laugh with this child as you think back over your adventures, and then together move forward as a team to find solutions that allow you to celebrate the wonderful person that you are.

About the Author

My professional career can be divided into two distinct segments. Prior to moving to Sioux Falls, South Dakota, in 2006, I enjoyed a thriving private practice as a clinical psychologist in northern Michigan. I specialized in the assessment of Attention Deficit/Hyperactivity Disorder, learning disabilities, and mood disorders, and was honored to have a large and loyal referral network that spanned the upper half of the state. I provided in-services on issues related to AD/HD for various agencies, gatherings, and organizations, including school districts, medical conferences, drug and alcohol treatment centers, and regional pharmacy conventions. I also was an adjunct faculty member at North Central Michigan College in the early 1990s.

Much of my professional work involves report writing, and I passionately believe in creating reports that bring each client to life, highlighting and integrating their special strengths, weaknesses, idiosyncrasies, and unique gifts.

During the summer of 2006, I moved with my husband and children to Sioux Falls so that my husband could join a rapidly expanding medical community. Taking advantage of this break in my own career, I decided to summarize in book form the knowledge that I had gained from evaluating AD/HD adults, which I believed I could do within a few months! One year later, I reemerged with a completed manuscript and a newfound respect for the trials and tribulations of aspiring writers!

In the fall of 2008, I reopened my private practice in Sioux Falls, and once again I am focusing on psychoeducational testing. As I meet and talk to adults with lifelong attentional struggles, I am able to put into context the difficulties that they have experienced, and I am struck by the heartfelt expressions of gratitude that I receive at the end of each session. Yet I recognize that there are a large number of undiagnosed AD/HD adults who berate themselves on a daily basis for their symptoms of inattention and impulsivity. It is my hope that this book will provide insight, education, and encouragement to this unique group of individuals.

Helpful Resources

Having AD/HD myself, I tend to gravitate to books that are compelling, informative, and not overly repetitive. (There is nothing worse than struggling through a paragraph, only to discover that the author is repeating a point that he or she already made.) Books that maintained my interest from start to finish include the following:

Ratey and Hallowell's *Driven to Distraction, Answers to Distraction,* and *Delivered from Distraction* are all highly recommended for AD/HD teens and adults.

Chris Zeigler Dendy offers a highly readable and well-organized book for AD/HD teens and their parents entitled *Teaching Teens with ADD and ADHD.*

Russell Barkley, in *Taking Charge of ADHD: The Complete, Authoritative Guide for Parents,* offers a helpful perspective on parenting children with AD/HD.

Jonathan Halverstadt, in *A.D.D. and Romance,* offers very interesting insights into relationships where one or both partners have AD/HD.

Recommended books written explicitly for women with attentional deficits include Sari Solden's *Women with Attention Deficit Disorder* and Kathleen Nadeau's *Understanding Girls with AD/HD.*

These books have been found to be helpful in the home setting:

- Judith Kolberg and Dr. Kathleen Nadeau's *ADD-Friendly Ways to Organize Your Life*
- Terry Matlen's *Survival Tips for Women with AD/HD: Beyond Piles, Palms, & Post-its*
- Deniece Schofield's *Confessions of an Organized Homemaker*

Eileen Bailey's website, *About ADD/ADHD,* is high on helpful household hints and low on guilt-inducing suggestions, and can be found at: http://add.about.com.

FlyLady.net (www.flylady.net) is another excellent and humorous online resource that provides daily tips on how to better organize your home and life.

ADDvance magazine, edited by Drs. Kathleen Nadeau and Patricia Quinn, offers a wide range of information for both men and women with AD/HD across the lifespan, and can be found at www.addvance .com.

Bibliography

Aase, Heidi, and Terje Sagvolden. "Moment-to-Moment Dynamics of ADHD Behaviour." *Behavioral and Brain Functions* 1 (2005):1–12.

Amen, Daniel. *Healing ADD.* New York: G. P. Putnam's Sons, 2001.

Barkley, Russell. *Attention-Deficit Hyperactivity Disorder: A Handbook for Diagnosis and Treatment.* New York: Guilford Press, 1998.

Barkley, Russell. *Attention-Deficit Hyperactivity Disorder: A Handbook for Diagnosis and Treatment* (3rd ed.). New York: Guilford Press, 2006.

Barkley, Russell. "Major Life Activity and Health Outcomes Associated with Attention-Deficit/Hyperactivity Disorder." *Journal of Clinical Psychiatry* 63 (2002): 10–15.

Barkley, Russell. *Taking Charge of ADHD, Revised Edition: The Complete, Authoritative Guide for Parents.* New York: Guilford Publications, 2002.

Barkley, Russell, George DuPaul, and Mary McMurray. "A Comprehensive Evaluation of Attention Deficit Disorder with and without Hyperactivity." *Journal of Consulting and Clinical Psychology* 58 (1990): 775–789.

Barkley, Russell, and Kevin Murphy. *Attention-Deficit Hyperactivity Disorder: A Clinical Workbook* (2nd ed.). New York: Guilford Press, 1998.

Barkley, Russell, Kevin Murphy, and Denise Kwasnik. "Motor Vehicle Driving Competencies and Risks in Teens and Young Adults with Attention Deficit Hyperactivity Disorder." *Pediatrics* 98 (1996): 1089–1095.

Bauermeister, Jose, Maribel Matos, Graciela Reins, Carmen Salas, Jose Martinez, Edward Cumba, et al. "Comparison of the DSM-IV Combined and Inattentive Types of ADHD in a School-Based Sample of Latino/Hispanic Children." *Journal of Child Psychology and Psychiatry* 46 (2005): 166–179.

Biederman, Joseph, Stephen Faraone, Eric Mick, Sarah Williamson, Timothy Wilens, Thomas Spencer, et al. "Clinical Correlates of AD/HD in Females: Findings from a Large Group of Girls Ascertained from Pediatric and Psychiatric Referral Services." *Journal of the American Academy of Child and Adolescent Psychiatry* 38 (1999): 966–975.

Biederman, Joseph, Anne Kwon, Megan Aleardi, Virginie-Anne Chouinard, Teresa Marino, Heather Cole, et al. "Absence of Gender Effects on Attention Deficit/Hyperactivity Disorder: Findings on Nonreferred Subjects." *The American Journal of Psychiatry* 162 (2005): 1083–1089.

Biederman, Joseph, Eric Mick, Stephen Faraone, Ellen Braaten, Alysa Doyle, Timothy Spencer, et al. "Influence of Gender on Attention Deficit Hyperactivity Disorder in Children Referred to a Psychiatric Clinic." *The American Journal of Psychiatry* 159 (2002): 36–42.

Biederman, Joseph, Carter Petty, Ronna Fried, Jessie Fontanella, Alysa Doyle, Larry Seidman, et al. "Impact of Psychometrically Defined Deficits of Executive Functioning in Adults with Attention Deficit Hyperactivity Disorder." *The American Journal of Psychiatry* 163 (2006): 1730–1738.

Brown, Thomas. "New Understanding of Attention Deficit Disorders in Children, Adolescents, and Adults: Assessment and Treatment." *Focus: The Official Newsletter of the National Attention Deficit Disorder Association (1999).*

Chhabildas, Nomita, Bruce Pennington, and Erik Willcutt. "A Comparison of the Neuropsychological Profiles of the DSM-IV Subtypes of ADHD." *Journal of Abnormal Child Development* 29 (2001): 529–540.

Crystal, David, Rick Ostrander, Ru San Chen, and Gerald August. "Multimethod Assessment of Psychopathology Among DSM-IV Subtypes of Children with Attention-Deficit/Hyperactivity Disorder: Self-, Parent, and Teacher Reports–Statistical Data Included." *Journal of Abnormal Child Psychology* 29 (2001): 189–205.

Diamond, Adele. "Attention-Deficit Disorder (Attention-Deficit/ Hyperactivity Disorder without Hyperactivity): A Neurobiologically and Behaviorally Distinct Disorder from Attention-Deficit/Hyperactivity Disorder (with

Hyperactivity)." *Development and Psychopathology* 17 (2005): 807–825.

Donnelly, Craig. "Defining Successful Pharmacologic Treatment of Attention Deficit Hyperactivity Disorder." *Behavioral Health Management* (May 2004).

Feld, Andrea, Charles Flatter, Kathryn Bernard, and Robert Brooks. "Resilience: Help Your Child Learn to Bounce Back." *Sesame Workshop* (June 7, 2007) http://www.sesameworkshop.org/parents/advice/article.php?contentId=80940&&.

Hallowell, Edward. "The Human Experience of ADD." Presented at the first national ADD conference for adults, "The Changing World of Adults with ADD," Ann Arbor, MI, 1993.

Hallowell, Edward and John Ratey. *Answers to Distractions.* New York: Pantheon Books, 1994.

Hallowell, Edward and John Ratey. *Delivered from Distraction: Getting the Most out of Life with Attention Deficit Disorder.* New York: Ballantine Books, 2005.

Hallowell, Edward and John Ratey. *Driven to Distraction.* New York: Simon & Schuster, 1994.

Halverstadt, Jonathan. *A.D.D. and Romance: Finding Fulfillment in Love, Sex, & Relationships.* Lanham: Taylor Trade Publishing, 1998.

Hartman, Christie, Eric Willcutt, Soo Hyun Rhee, and Bruce Pennington. "The Relation Between Sluggish Cognitive Tempo and DSM-IV ADHD." *Journal of Abnormal Child Psychology* 32 (2004): 491–503.

Hay, David. "Should Sluggish Cognitive Tempo Symptoms Be Included in the Diagnosis of Attention-Deficit/Hyperactivity Disorder?" *Journal of the American Academy of Child and Adolescent Psychiatry* 43 (2004): 588–597.

Kelly, Kate and Peggy Ramundo. *You Mean I'm Not Lazy, Stupid, or Crazy?* New York: Fireside, 1993.

Kennedy, Robert and Robert Glassman. "Subtypes in ADHD: A Newsmaker Interview with Mary Solanto, PhD." *Medscape Medical News.* (November 2006) http://www.medscape.com/viewarticle/463181.

Kohlberg, Judith and Kathleen Nadeau. *ADD-Friendly Ways to Organize Your Life.* New York: Brunner-Routledge, 2002.

Korn, Martin. "Treatment for Adult ADHD: A Newsmaker Interview with Timothy Wilens, MD." *Medscape Medical News.* (January 12, 2007) http://www.medscape.com/viewarticle/477487.

Levine, Mel. *One Mind at a Time.* New York: Simon & Schuster, 2002.

Levine, Mel. *Ready or Not, Here Life Comes.* New York: Simon & Schuster, 2005.

Matlen, Terry. *Survival Tips for Women with AD/HD: Beyond Piles, Palms, & Post-its.* Plantation, FL: Specialty Press, Inc., 2005.

McBurnett, Keith, Linda Pfiffner, and Paul Frick. "Symptom Properties as a Function of ADHD Type: An Argument for Continued Study of Sluggish Cognitive Tempo—Statistical Data Included." *Journal of Abnormal Child Psychology* 29 (2001): 207–213.

Milich, Richard, Amy Ballentine, and Donald Lynam. "ADHD Combined Type and ADHD Predominantly Inattentive Type are Distinct and Unrelated Disorders." *Clinical Psychology: Science and Practice* 8 (2001): 463–488.

Millstein, Rachael, Timothy Wilens, Joseph Biederman, and Thomas Spencer. "Presenting ADHD Symptoms and Subtypes in Clinically Referred Adults with ADHD." *Journal of Attention Disorders* 2 (1997): 159–166.

Murphy, Kevin and Russell Barkley. "Attention Deficit Hyperactivity Disorder in Adults." *Comprehensive Psychiatry* 37 (1996), 393–401.

Murphy, Kevin, Russell Barkley, and Tracie Bush. "Young Adults with Attention Deficit Hyperactivity Disorder: Subtype Differences in Comorbidity, Educational, and Clinical History." *The Journal of Nervous and Mental Disease* 190 (2002): 147–157.

Nadeau, Kathleen. "Feeling Overwhelmed, Disorganized, Scattered?" *ADDvance: A Magazine for Women with Attention Deficit Disorder.* (March 14, 2007) http://www.add.org/articles/overwhelmed.html.

Nadeau, Kathleen, Ellen Littman, and Patricia Quinn. *Understanding Girls with AD/HD.* Washington, D.C.: Advantage Books, 1999.

Nadeau, Kathleen and Patricia Quinn. *Understanding Women with AD/HD.* Washington, D.C.: Advantage Books, 2002.

Nadeau, Kathleen and Patricia Quinn. "Women and AD/HD." *Attention Deficit Disorder Association.* (March 14, 2007) http://www.add.org/articles/womenadhd.html.

Nigg, Joel, Lisa Blaskey, Cynthia Huang-Pollock, and Marsha Rappley. "Neuropsychological Executive Functions and DSM-IV ADHD Subtypes." *Journal of the American Academy of Child and Adolescent Psychiatry* 41 (2002): 59–66.

Nigg, Joel, Stephen Hinshaw, and Cynthia Huang-Pollock. "Disorders of Attention and Impulse Regulation." *Developmental Psychopathology, Vol. 3: Risk, Disorder, and Adaptation* (2nd ed.), edited by Dante Cicchetti and Donald Cohen. New York: John Wiley & Sons, 2006.

Purvis, Karen and Rosemary Tannock. "Language Abilities in Children with Attention Deficit Hyperactivity Disorder, Reading Disabilities, and Normal Controls." *Journal of Abnormal Child Psychology* 25 (2004): 133–144.

Quinn, Patricia and Kathleen Nadeau. *When Moms and Kids Have ADD (ADHD).* Washington D.C.: Advantage Books, 2005.

Robins, Arthur. *ADHD in Adolescents.* New York: Guilford Press, 1998.

Robins, Arthur. "Can Your Marriage Survive AD/HD?" *Attention! The Magazine for Families and Adults with Attention-Deficit/Hyperactivity Disorder* (June 2001).

Seidman, Larry, Joseph Biederman, Michael Monuteaux, Eve Valera, Alysa Doyle, and Stephen Faraone. "Impact of Gender and Age on Executive Functioning: Do Girls and Boys with and without Attention Deficit Hyperactivity Disorder Differ Neuropsychologically in Preteen and Teenage Years?" *Developmental Neuropsychology* 27 (2005): 79–105.

Schofield, Deniece. *Confessions of an Organized Homemaker.* Cincinnati, OH: Betterway Books, 1994.

Sogn, Richard. "AD/HD Medications and Treatments." *WebMD* (2006) http://blogs.webmd.com/adhdmedicationsandtreatments.

Solden, Sari. *Women with Attention Deficit Disorder.* Nevada City, CA: Underwood Books, 1995.

Sussman, Norman. "In Session with Richard H. Weisler, MD: Treatment of Attention-Deficit/Hyperactivity Disorder." *Primary Psychiatry* 14 (2007): 39–42.

Turnock, Patrick, Lee Rosen, and Patricia Kaminski. "Difference in Academic Coping Strategies of College Students who Self-Report High and Low Symptoms of Attention Deficit Hyperactivity Disorder." *Journal of College Student Development* (Sep/Oct 1998) http://findarticles.com/p/articles/mi_qa3752/is_199809/.../pg_5/.

Watkins, Carol. "ADD in the Home." *Attention Deficit Disorder Association* (2007) http://www.add.org/articles/women.html.

Weiss, Lynn. *A.D.D. on the Job: Making Your A.D.D. Work for You.* Dallas: Taylor Publishing Company, 1996.

Weiss, Lynn. *A.D.D. & Success.* Dallas: Taylor Publishing Company, 1998.

Weiss, Lynn. *Attention Deficit Disorder in Adults: A Different Way of Thinking* (4th ed.). Dallas: Taylor Publishing Company, 2005.

Wender, Paul. *Attention-Deficit Hyperactivity Disorder in Adults.* New York: Oxford University Press, 1988.

Zeigler Dendy, Chris. *Teaching Teens with ADD and ADHD.* Bethesda, MD: Woodbine House, Inc., 2000.

Notes

Chapter 1

[1]. Edward Hallowell, "The Human Experience of ADD" (keynote speaker at the first national ADD conference for adults, "The Changing World of Adults with ADD," Ann Arbor, Michigan, 1993).

Chapter 2

[2]. Edward Hallowell and John Ratey, *Driven to Distraction* (New York: Simon & Schuster, 1994).

[3]. Studies have consistently shown that ADHD adolescents and young adults are at much higher risk for traffic citations (particularly for speeding), repeated car accidents, and crashes that result in bodily injury than their non-AD/HD cohorts (Barkley 2006). In addition, AD/HD drivers are more likely than non-AD/HD drivers to be rated by themselves and by their passengers as having unsafe driving habits, such as erratic steering, false breaking, and slow reaction times (Barkley et al. 1996).

[4]. Heidi Aase and Terje Sagvolden, "Moment to Moment Dynamics of ADHD Behaviour," *Behavior and Brain Function* 1 (2005): 1–12.

[5]. Russell Barkley, *Attention-Deficit Hyperactivity Disorder: A Handbook for Diagnosis and Treatment* (New York: Guilford Press, 2006).

[6]. Further discussion of hyperfocus can be found in Chapter 5, "The Gift and the Curse of Hyperfocus."

Chapter 3

[7]. Edward Hallowell and John Ratey, *Driven to Distraction* (New York: Simon & Schuster, 1994), 74.

[8]. Sari Solden discusses the feeling of "paralysis" when overwhelmed, in her 1995 book, W*omen with Attention Deficit Disorders: Embrace Your Differences and Transform Your Life.*

Chapter 4

[9]. Edward Hallowell and John Ratey, *Driven to Distraction* (New York: Simon & Schuster, 1994).

[10]. Larry Seidman et al., "Impact of Gender and Age on Executive Functioning: Do Girls and Boys with and without Attention Deficit Hyperactivity Disorder Differ Neuropsychologically in Preteen and Teenage Years?" *Developmental Neuropsychology* 27 (2005): 79–105.

[11]. Thomas Brown, "New Understanding of Attention Deficit Disorders in Children, Adolescents, and Adults: Assessment and Treatment." *Focus: The Official Newsletter of the National Attention Deficit Disorder Association* (1999).

[12]. Working memory is the process of actively manipulating information that is stored in short-term memory (for example, when computing mathematical operations in one's head). This cognitive function is easily disrupted by distractions and therefore is a particular weakness for those with AD/HD.

[13]. Joseph Biederman et al., "Clinical Correlates of AD/HD in Females: Findings from a Large Group of Girls Ascertained from Pediatric and Psychiatric Referral Services." *Journal of the American Academy of Child and Adolescent Psychiatry* 38 (1999): 966–975.

[14]. For a thorough list of recommendations, Eileen Bailey's informative Web site, *About ADD/ADHD*, is highly recommended and can be found at: http://add.about.com/cs/addthebasics/a/communication.htm.

Chapter 5

[15]. Edward Hallowell and John Ratey, *Driven to Distraction* (New York: Simon & Schuster, 1994).

[16]. Other terms that have been used to describe this state are *overfocus* and *flow.*

[17]. Hallowell and Ratey, in *Answers to Distractions,* described the state of hyperfocus (or "flow") as "a time when we are so involved in what we are doing that we forget our worries, our concerns, our bills, our cavities, our enemies, our cravings, and we join our project so completely that we become it for a while."

Chapter 8

[18]. Transitioning from one activity to another is particularly difficult for children with AD/HD, and the literature is replete with recommendations on how to assist children during such times. "Give the AD/HD child a five-minute warning" is advice commonly offered to parents to prepare their child for an upcoming transition and to avoid emotional meltdowns that may otherwise occur when the AD/HD child is expected to shift his or her focus from one activity (watching cartoons) to the next (getting ready for dinner). This difficulty is not necessarily due to the AD/HD children's reluctance to stop an activity in which he or she is engaged. In fact, parents speak in bewildered tones about temper tantrums that their AD/HD child has thrown when getting ready for an enjoyable outing that the child has been looking forward to all day. What they are witnessing may well be the AD/HD child's negative response to the increased stimulation that is inherent in any activity change.

[19]. In my practice, less than one-third of adults with AD/HD reported problems with anger management.

[20]. The heritability of AD/HD refers to the extent to which genetics influences the likelihood of developing AD/HD.

[21]. Sari Solden, *Women with Attention Deficit Disorder* (Nevada City, CA: Underwood Books, 1995).

[22]. Although I have enjoyed the benefits of stimulant medication for the past fifteen years, and have seen a huge improvement in my ability to parent in a purposeful, goal-oriented manner, I broach this topic with great trepidation, knowing that I may be branded by some as a pill-pushing heretic who merely wants to drug the livelier members of our society into a state of stuporous submission. Given the overwhelming evidence as to the benefits of stimulant medication for a substantial percentage of AD/HD individuals, I find it absolutely amazing that these findings can be refuted by fringe organizations that provide no credible scientific evidence to support their counter claims. I am equally incredulous over the typical media coverage of this issue, which often gives equal weight to alternative perspectives, regardless of the credentials of the respondents.

[23]. An approach advocated by Dr. Russell Barkley in *Taking Charge of ADHD, Revised Edition: The Complete, Authoritative Guide for Parents.*

[24]. Mel Levine, *Ready or Not, Here Life Comes* (New York: Simon & Schuster, 2005), 7.

[25]. Andrea Feld et al., "Resilience: Help Your Child Learn to Bounce Back," *Sesame Workshop* (June 7, 2007) http://www.sesameworkshop.org/parents/advice/article.php?contentId=80940&&.

Chapter 13

[26]. Joel Nigg et al. suggest that the relatively late maturation of executive functioning may account in part for AD/HD's changing presentation in adolescence and adulthood.

[27]. Edward Hallowell and John Ratey, *Delivered from Distraction: Getting the Most out of Life with Attention Deficit Disorder* (New York: Ballantine Books, 2005), 22.

[28]. One goal of a thorough psychological evaluation is to determine whether self-reports of anxiety represent an anxiety disorder independent of AD/HD, whether this perceived anxiety is misinterpreted symptoms of internal restlessness, or whether the reported anxiety is secondary (or in response) to the problems associated with AD/HD.

[29]. Martin Korn, "Treatment for Adult ADHD: A Newsmaker Interview with Timothy Wilens, MD." *Medscape Medical News.* (2004) http://www.medscape.com/viewarticle/477487.

[30]. Ibid.

[31]. Edward Hallowell and John Ratey, *Driven to Distraction* (New York: Simon & Schuster, 1994), 173.

[32]. Craig Donnelly, "Defining Successful Pharmacologic Treatment of Attention Deficit Hyperactivity Disorder," *Behavioral Health Management* (May 2004).

Chapter 14

[33]. By the end of the decade there were over two thousand published studies on this topic, a number that has since tripled (Barkley 2006).

[34]. Diagnostic and Statistical Manual of Mental Disorders–Third Edition

[35]. These diagnostic terms have since been changed—twice, in fact—and currently we use the term *Attention Deficit/Hyperactivity Disorder–Combined type* to refer to those individuals with symptoms of both hyperactivity and inattention, and *AD/HD–Predominantly Inattentive subtype* to refer to persons who display predominant features of inattention but few or no symptoms of hyperactivity. There is also a third subtype, *AD/HD–Predominantly Hyperactive-Impulsive,* but there is increasing evidence to suggest that this subtype represents younger hyperactive children who have not yet developed symptoms of inattention, and who

ultimately will meet the criteria for AD/HD–Combined type.

[36]. According to a community-based study completed by Dr. Joseph Biederman and his colleagues in 2005, 25 percent of girls and 27 percent of boys meet the criteria for the predominantly inattentive subgroup.

[37]. This subset is estimated by Dr. Russell Barkley to account for 30–50 percent of the inattentive subtype (Barkley 2006).

[38]. Russell Barkley, *Attention-Deficit Hyperactivity Disorder: A Handbook for Diagnosis and Treatment* (New York: Guilford Press, 2006).

[39]. Kevin Murphy et al., "Young Adults with Attention Deficit Hyperactivity Disorder: Subtype Differences in Comorbidity, Educational, and Clinical History," *The Journal of Nervous and Mental Disease* 190 (2002): 147–157.

[40]. Russell Barkley, 2006; Jose Bauermeister et al., 2005; Adele Diamond, 2005; Richard Milich et al., 2001.

[41]. Nomita Chhabildas et al., 2001; Joel Nigg et al., 2006.

[42]. For particularly intense clients or for those with a history of mood swings, the possibility of a bipolar disorder is explored as well.

[43]. Modified adult thresholds, recommended by Dr. Russell Barkley (2006), were utilized to determine whether or not an adult met the DSM-IV criteria for AD/HD. These thresholds identify those adults whose symptoms are more severe than 93 percent of his or her same-age peers.

[44]. Table 1: Summary of Presenting Symptoms of AD/HD-C (in bold print) and AD-HD-PI by age group

	Total	18–24	25–44	45–65
Sustained attention	**77%**	**81%**	**81%**	**67%**
	80%	86%	89%	59%
Restlessness	**73%****	**77%****	**73%****	**69%****
	20%	10%	28%	29%
Disorganization	**61%**	**66%**	**58%**	**58%**
	67%	62%	72%	71%
Easily distracted	**56%**	**58%**	**52%**	**60%****
	48%	62%	50%	24%
Reading retention problems	**44%**	**64%**	**29%**	**48%**
	48%	62%	33%	41%
Impulsivity	**34%****	**43%****	**30%**	**31%**
	13%	3%	22%	18%
Forgetful in activities	**33%**	**34%**	**33%**	**31%**
	38%	45%	39%	24%
Anger management problems	**29%**	**32%****	**34%**	**17%**
	16%	3%	22%	29%
Inattention to detail/careless errors	**29%**	**47%**	**24%**	**19%**
	30%	45%	22%	12%
Academic/Work Underachievement	**21%**	**28%**	**22%**	**10%**
	31%	49%	17%	24%
Procrastination	**21%**	**32%**	**15%**	**19%**
	25%	38%	22%	6%
Overwhelmed	**19%**	**11%**	**22%**	**23%**
	41%**	28%	67%**	35%
Doesn't listen when others talk	**18%**	**13%**	**23%**	**17%**
	16%	24%	11%	6%
Misplaces/loses items	**14%**	**13%**	**11%**	**19%**
	20%	3%	39%**	29%
Communication problems	**12%**	**19%**	**10%**	**8%**
	23%*	21%	28%	24%
Time management problems	**12%**	**13%**	**11%**	**13%**
	17%	14%	33%	6%
Poor follow through requests	**7%**	**17%**	**3%**	**2%**
	17%*	28%	11%	6%

**significant at .01 level   *significant at .05 level

[45]. To illustrate these similarities, presenting problems that were mentioned *with equal frequency* by the inattentive and combined subgroups are listed below, along with illustrative statements from members of each subtype.

Sustained attention

- "I'll be sitting and talking with someone and just drift off, totally lose concentration."
- "When sitting in staff meetings I find myself daydreaming and will have no idea what is being said."

Disorganization

- "I try to organize my work area, but within a short period of time my workspace is a big cluttered mess."
- "I have piles of papers all over the surface of my desk."

Reading Retention Problems

- "I have to read material several times before it sticks."
- "I can read a page over and over and still miss the main point of the text."

Distractibility

- "I'm easily distracted by noises on the job and will often stop what I am doing and investigate what's going on."
- "I am easily distracted, especially during tests, and if anyone makes the slightest noise I lose my train of thought."

Forgetfulness

- "I will go to my truck at least ten to fifteen times during the day to get a particular tool, but by the time I get there, I've already forgotten what it was that I needed."
- "If given more than one thing to do at a time, I often end up forgetting part of the instructions."

Academic/Work Underachievement

- "I would like to go back to school to be trained for a more challenging profession, but I don't have the concentration skills."
- "I realized a while ago that although I want to do well, I don't seem to be able to do so."

Inattention to Detail/Careless Errors

- "I frequently overlook details, and going back to correct them takes up extra time during my day."
- "I make mistakes on daily forms that I'm required to fill out."

Misplacing/Losing Items

- "I lose track of anything I'm supposed to keep track of."
- "When I work on a project, I put down my tools and then am unable to locate them when I need them next."

Poor Task Persistence

- "I always have good intentions, but I never get anything accomplished. I have projects all over the house that have been started, but by nighttime nothing is finished."
- "My house is in total chaos because of the many unfinished projects that exist."

Procrastination

- "I often wait until the last minute to do an assignment."
- "I have particular problems doing paperwork, and I put it off until it's reached a crisis proportion."

Time Management Problems

- "Allotting time for my daily tasks is very difficult for me."
- "I have a poor sense of passing time, and as a result I'm often late for appointments."

[46]. Forty-three percent of young adults with AD/HD–Combined form presented with symptoms of impulsivity, as compared to only 3 percent of young adults with the inattentive type of AD/HD. Relatedly, whereas 30 percent of the combined group in the youngest age bracket mentioned problems with anger management, only 3 percent of the inattentive subgroup in this age bracket found anger control to be an issue.

[47]. Carol Watkins, "ADD in the Home," *Attention Deficit Disorder Association* (2007) http://www.add.org/articles/women.html.

[48]. Among male respondents, 27 percent of the inattentive subgroup reported feeling overwhelmed, while only 8 percent of males in the combined group reported this difficulty. Among female respondents, 59 percent of the inattentive subgroup reported feeling overwhelmed, whereas 28 percent of women in the combined subtype noted such problems.

[49]. A whopping 82 percent of predominantly inattentive women in this age bracket reported feeling overwhelmed, while 29 percent of women from the combined subtype reported such problems. (Forty-three percent of inattentive men in this age group reported feeling overwhelmed as compared to 12 percent of men in the combined subtype. This latter finding was not, however, statistically significant—arguably due to the small sample size.)

Chapter 15

[50]. According to Nadeau, Littman, & Quinn, authors of *Understanding Girls with AD/HD*, a worsening of AD/HD symptoms may be observed in girls at the time of puberty. Hallowell and Ratey in *Answers to Distraction* note that behavioral problems in females often appear to coincide with the onset of puberty.

[51]. Kathleen Nadeau and Patricia Quinn, 2002; Norman Sussman, 2007; Richard Sogn, 2006.

[52]. Martin Korn, "Treatment for Adult ADHD: A Newsmaker Interview with Timothy Wilens, MD." *Medscape Medical News.* (2004) http://www.medscape.com/viewarticle/477487.

[53]. Russell Bartley, 2006; Kathleen Nadeau and Patricia Quinn, 2002; Paul Wender, 1988.

[54]. Patrick Turnock et al., "Difference in Academic Coping Strategies of College Students who Self-Report High and Low Symptoms of Attention Deficit Hyperactivity Disorder," *Journal of College Student Development* (Sep/Oct 1998).

Chapter 16

[55]. Sari Solden, *Women with Attention Deficit Disorder* (Nevada City, CA: Underwood Books, 1995), 55.